PROFESSIONS - TRAINING, EDUCATION AND DEMOGRAPHICS

# THE FAMILY DOCTORS

# IMAGES AND METAPHORS OF THE FAMILY DOCTOR TO LEARN FAMILY MEDICINE

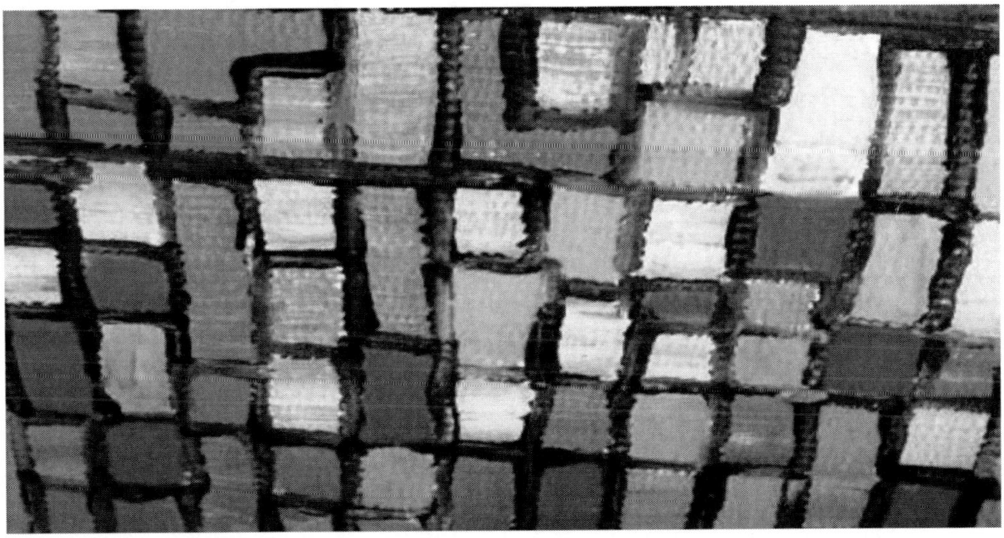

# PROFESSIONS - TRAINING, EDUCATION AND DEMOGRAPHICS

Additional books in this series can be found on Nova's website
under the Series tab.

Additional eBooks in this series can be found on Nova's website
under the eBooks tab.

PROFESSIONS - TRAINING, EDUCATION AND DEMOGRAPHICS

# THE FAMILY DOCTORS

## IMAGES AND METAPHORS OF THE FAMILY DOCTOR TO LEARN FAMILY MEDICINE

JOSÉ LUIS TURABIAN
AND
BENJAMIN PEREZ-FRANCO

New York

Additional color graphics may be available in the e-book version of this book.

**Library of Congress Cataloging-in-Publication Data**

Names: Turabiban, Josbe Luis, editor. | Pberez Franco, Benjambin, editor.
Title: The family doctors : images and metaphors of the family doctor to learn family medicine / editors, Josbe Luis Turabian and Benjamin Perez-Franco (Medico de Familia, Tutor de Residentes, Centro de Salud Poligono Industrial, SESCAM, Toledo, Spain, and others).
Description: Hauppauge, New York : Nova Science Publisher's, Inc., [2016] | Includes index. | Description based on print version record and CIP data provided by publisher; resource not viewed.
Identifiers: LCCN 2016019638 (print) | LCCN 2016017055 (ebook) | ISBN 9781634852074 () | ISBN 9781634851763 (hardcover) | ISBN 9781634852074 (ebook)
Subjects: LCSH: Family medicine. | Primary care (Medicine)
Classification: LCC RC46 (print) | LCC RC46 .F34 2016 (ebook) | DDC 610--dc23 LC record available at https://lccn.loc.gov/2016019638

*Published by Nova Science Publishers, Inc. † New York*

# Contents

# Preface

Medicine is often learned through a mechanistic metaphor of biology and a military metaphor of war. However, the conceptual elements and skills that promote the mastery of family medicine, such as contextual knowledge, continuity of care, the clinical interview, comprehensiveness, coordination, and so on, are often difficult to explain and to understand. Furthermore, these fundamental concepts of family medicine have nothing to do with the metaphor of the machine or the metaphor of war. In this book, these concepts are explained through metaphors that are more explanatory, nicer, sweeter, and more playful. Thinking based on metaphors and comparisons is a way of making a concept so suggestive, interesting and surprising that it reaches people more easily.

The value of family medicine lies in its distinctiveness from academic medicine; it is a unique discipline that defines itself in terms of relationships, especially those between the doctor and patient. Family physicians tend to think in terms of individual patients rather than of abstractions and generalizations, and family medicine is based more on the metaphor of an organism rather than that of mechanistic biology. Family medicine is unique in the medical arena in that it transcends the duality of body and mind. Thus, the family doctor should be encouraged to use a non-conventional form when thinking about the problems that are presented in the consultation (for example, thinking on the basis of metaphors).

*Chapter 1*

# Introduction

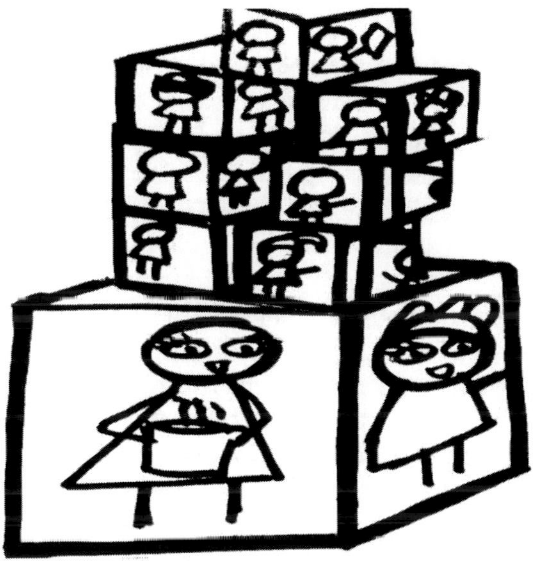

The family doctor is the general practitioner who assumes professional responsibility for attention to the whole patient, not selecting according to undifferentiated problems, and who has committed himself to the person independent of age, sex, disease, organs or corporal systems.

The clinical specialty of family medicine focuses on the patient. It is based on evidence, centered on the family, and orientated to the problem. Family physicians acquire and maintain a wide range of skills that depend on the needs of the patients and the communities they serve. The scope of their practice is not defined by diagnoses or procedures, but by human needs.

Family physicians do not treat diseases; they take care of people. The nodal points in the life cycle of the family, such as birth, severe illness, and end of life, deserve special attention.

Family physicians are experts in the management of common problems, recognizing the important diseases, discovering hidden conditions, and managing acute and chronic diseases.

Family physicians emphasize health promotion and disease prevention. Their knowledge, skills, and attitudes are directed to the practice community, and are based on current scientific knowledge and focused on the continuous improvement in quality.

Family practice requires special skills to be able to identify concerns, negotiate plans and help to solve problems. The recognition, integration and prioritization of multiple concerns and the synthesis of solutions are critical clinical competencies.

The wide variety of human needs requires the guidance of clinical processes, shared responsibility, and the management of uncertainty. A focus on the person requires observation skills, communication skills, and understanding.

Family medicine is, first and foremost, a speciality of primary care and primary health care is expanding and becoming much more complex in this new era of information systems.

However, family physicians are not a conglomerate of miniature versions of paediatricians, internists and psychiatrists, but are specialists in their own right, with their own borders and specialist content.

The academic discipline of family medicine is unique and coherent. It has a core of knowledge, skills and attitudes that are common to all clinical specialities, and to other specialities in community medicine, the behavioural sciences and the social sciences. However, family medicine uses them in a unique way, applying them to their own contexts and thus constituting a recognizable unitary and specific, differentiated set of skills.

Thus, although the work of the family doctor is enormous — encompassing the areas of paediatrics, internal medicine, and psychiatry, and most of the remaining medical specialties — its methods and working tools are different or overlap with those used by specialists in related fields.

The conceptual elements of family medicine and the skills that promote its mastery are "material" (methods/processes), used as bricks to construct the building of family medicine (context, continuity, interview, comprehensiveness, coordination, etc.). These conceptual materials have real value: the building may be destroyed but the materials used retains their value, and these are the foundations of family medicine, although they are also applied in other specialist fields in accordance with their own methods.

Therefore, it is logical that the concepts and theories that belonging to family medicine are often difficult to explain and to understand. In this book, these concepts are explained through metaphors.

Metaphors enable us to understand something that is unknown in terms of its familiarity. For this reason, they are used frequently in all sciences that adopt common words to name complex realities. The metaphors are analogue devices, used to illuminate reality.

Metaphors can simplify expert knowledge, not by ignoring or reducing the inherent complexity, but by providing a point of entry for its comprehension. They are a means of generating ideas, promoting creativity, and constructing concepts and theories.

Thinking based on metaphors and comparisons is a way of transforming a concept into something that is so suggestive, interesting, and surprising, that it reaches people more easily.

In this book, we chose certain words and images that have a metaphorical dimension in the field of family medicine. They have been chosen for their capacity to compare the tasks of the family doctor and to allow us to gain a better understanding of his or her work.

Medicine is often learned as a mechanistic metaphor (based on the machine) of biology. It is also accompanied by a military metaphor of war.

The disease is a war: inflammation is the battle against germs and the battle is lost if the germs win the infection. It is immunity that expires in battle. The disease is described in terms of a battle engaged in the nineteenth century. The bacteria invade and leukocytes strike. These are images of romantic battles, British troops attacking the army of the Caliph, killing three of the British and thousands of dervishes while the British commander observes the great victory through field glasses.

The drugs are understood through the metaphor of "magic bullets."

Medical education can be understood through a military metaphor: hierarchies, ranges, structures (department head, tutors); uniforms (robes, pyjamas); and training to be in the firing line (always working between life and death, the call at three in the morning like a walk through a minefield). The professor who teaches the medical students has been in war and has learnt from the experience.

In family medicine, however, these mechanistic or military metaphors are neither useful nor desirable. They are metaphors that do not correspond to the fundamental conceptual basis of family medicine. Living organisms have properties that are not machines: they grow, regenerate, heal, learn, and organize themselves. An organism is particularly complex and uncertain.

In this book "the true metaphors of family medicine" are displayed. The fundamental concepts of family medicine are explained through other metaphors, ones that are more explanatory, nicer, sweeter, and more playful.

The value of family medicine lies in its difference from academic medicine. It is a unique discipline that defines itself in terms of relations, especially the relations between the doctor and the patient, and family physicians tend to think in terms of individual patients rather than in abstractions and generalizations. Family medicine is based more on the metaphor of an organism that it is on a metaphor of a mechanistic biology and it is unique as an area of medicine that transcends the duality of body and mind.

Therefore, the family doctor should be encouraged to think about the problems that are presented in the consultation in a non-conventional form, for example, on the basis of metaphors.

The majority of family physicians are women, so "the feminine" of the family doctor is a fundamental aspect.

The chapters of this book present some images or metaphors of the family doctor. Certainly the concepts that incorporate these images can, on occasions, partly overlap but we think that this fact helps to understand the fundamental concepts of family medicine.

## References

AAFP. "Family Medicine, Definition of." http://www.aafp.org/online/en/home/policy/policies/f/fammeddef.html.

AAFP. "Family Medicine, Scope and Philosophical Statement." http://www.aafp.org/online/en/home/policy/policies/f/scopephil.html.

Berger J. A fortunate man. New York: Vintage Books. Random House, Inc; 1997.

Casper ST, Welsh R. British Romantic Generalism in the Age of Specialism, 1870–1990. *Soc Hist Med.* 2016; 29 (1): 154-174. http://shm.oxfordjournals.org/content/29/1/154.full?etoc.

Conn JJ. What can clinical teachers learn from Harry Potter and the Philosopher's Stone?, *Medical Education.* 2002; 36(12): 1176-1181. http://www.blackwell-synergy.com/links/doi/10.1046/j.1365-2923.2002.01376.x.

González Blasco P. Literature and Movies for Medical Students. *Fam Med.* 2001; 33(6):426-8. http://www.sobramfa.com.br/artigos/2001_jun_literature_and_movies_for_medical_students.pdf.

De Bono E. Wordpower. Bungay, Suffolk; Richard Clay (The Chaucer Press) Ltd; 1977.

Dolev JC, Friedlaender LK, Braverman IM. Use of Fine Art to Enhance Visual Diagnostic Skills. *JAMA.* 2001;286(9):1020-1021. http://jama.jamanetwork.com/article.aspx?articleid=1031468.

Fabb WE, Chao DVK, Chan CSY. The trouble with family medicine - *Fam Pract.* 1997; 14(1): 5-11. http://fampra.oxfordjournals.org/content/14/1/5.full.pdf.

Gómez de la Serna R. Greguerías. Madrid: Castalia; 1994.

Gómez de la Serna R. Nuevas páginas de mi vida. Madrid: Alianza Editorial; 1970.

Hurwitz B. Narrative and the practice of medicine. *Lancet* 2000;356:2086-89. http://www.thelancet.com/pdfs/journals/lancet/PIIS0140-6736(00)03412-7.pdf.

Milligan T. The physician as computer: a modern medical metaphor. *Fam Med.* 1998; 30(7): 480-1.

Operational Definitions of Attributes of Primary Health Care: Consensus Among Canadian Experts. *Annals of Family Medicine* 5:336-344 (2007). http://www.annfammed.org/cgi/content/full/5/4/336.

Pearson H. Doctors examine art. Art appreciation class improves student doctors' diagnosis. *Nature.* 2001. http://www.nature.com/nsu/010913/010913-11.html.

Phillips WR, Haynes DG. The domain of family practice: scope, role, and function. *Fam Med.* 2001;33(4):273-7. http://www.ncbi.nlm.nih.gov/pubmed/11322520.

Reisfield GM, Wilson GR. Use of Metaphor in the Discourse on Cancer. *Journal of Clinical Oncology.* http://jco.ascopubs.org/content/22/19/4024.full.

Skelton JR, Macleod JAA, Thomas CP. Teaching literature and medicine to medical students, part II: why literature and medicine?. *Lancet* 2000;356:2001-3. http://www.thelancet.com/pdfs/journals/lancet/PIIS0140-6736(00)03318-3.pdf.

Skelton JR, Thomas CP, Macleod JAA. Teaching literature and medicine to medical students, part I: the beginning. *Lancet* 2000;356:1920-2. http://www.thelancet.com/pdfs/journals/lancet/PIIS0140-6736(00)03270-0.pdf.

Skelton JR; Wearn AM; Hobbs FD. A concordance-based study of metaphoric expressions used by general practitioners and patients in consultation. *Br J Gen Pract* 2002;52(475):114-8. http://www.ncbi.nlm.nih.gov/pubmed/11887876.

Sontag S. Illness as metaphor. Aids and its metaphors. London: Penguin Books, 1991.

Turabian JL ¿Para qué servimos los médicos de familia? *JANO* 2006;1628:14, http://www.jano.es/ficheros/sumarios/1/0/1628/14/1v0n1628a13094844pdf001.pdf.

Turabian JL. Cuadernos de Medicina de Familia y Comunitaria. Una introducción a los principios de Medicina de Familia. Madrid: Díaz de Santos. 1995. http://www.amazon.co.uk/Cuadernos-medicina-familia-y-comunitaria/dp/8479781920.

Turabian JL. El misterioso caso del médico de familia. JANO 2007;1636:14. http://apps.elsevier.es/watermark/ctl_servlet?_f=10&pident_articulo=13098315&pident_usuario=0&pcontactid=&pident_revista=1&ty=57&accion=L&origen=elsevier&web=www.elsevier.es&lan=es&fichero=1v0n1636a13098315pdf001.pdf.

Wellbery C, McAteer RA. The Art of Observation: A Pedagogical Framework. *Acad Med.* 2015;90(12): 1624-30. http://www.ncbi.nlm.nih.gov/pubmed/26164640.

*Chapter 2*

# The Family Doctor as a Female Family Doctor

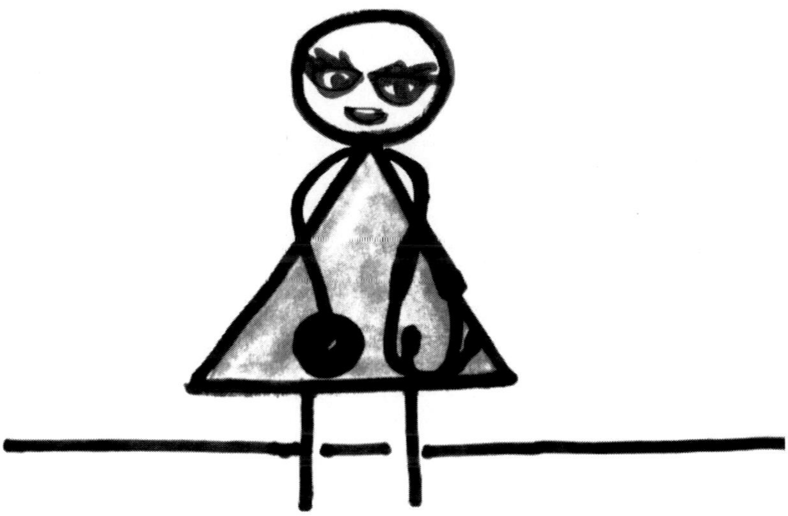

Females family doctors have consultation major skills in family medicine that may not be found in male doctors. Women identify emotionally with the stories of their patients, whereas the men remain more distant, seeing them as a source (fountain) of abstract facts. Thus female family doctors may demonstrate more genuine interest in the life story of the patient, exercising less control over the content of the interview. The female family doctor might also provide more integrated information to the patient, demonstrating greater empathy and devoting more time to them than the male doctor.

For male doctors, their professional satisfaction is the recognition on the part of his patients. For the female's doctors, the recognition of their patients means an affective link.

Females doctors perceive of something as important if it contributes positively or negatively to them reaching their goals, to their personal characteristics or internal attributions, such as their personality, their own expectations, their experience, their motivation and their control over situations and feelings. In contrast, male doctors are not in the habit of linking their achievements with their internal attributions but with their social recognition.

The skills of the female family doctor are not biologically innate but can be learned and practised by both females and males. What this means is that males family doctors need to be a bit more like female family doctors.

## References

Dahrouge S, Seale E, Hogg W, Russell G, Younger J, Muggah E, et al. A Comprehensive Assessment of Family Physician Gender and Quality of Care: A Cross-Sectional Analysis in Ontario, Canada. *Med Care.* 2016; [Epub ahead of print]. http://www.ncbi.nlm.nih.gov/pubmed/26765146.

Freeman J. Women in Family Medicine: Gender Diversity and Beyond. *Fam Med* 2011;43(3):153-4. https://www.stfm.org/fmhub/fm2011/March/Joshua153.pdf.

Howe A. Why family medicine benefits from more women doctors, - *Br J Gen Pract.* 2007; 57(535): 91–92. http://www.ncbi.nlm.nih.gov/pmc/articles/PMC2034165/.

Keuken DG, Haafkens JA, Hellema MJ, Burgers JS, Moerman CJ. Incorporating a gender perspective into the development of clinical guidelines: a training course for guideline developers. Implementation *Science.* 2007, 2:35. http://www.implementation science.com/content/2/1/35/abstract.

McCarthy M. Women make up majority of trainees in seven US specialties. *BMJ* 2015;351:h4614. http://www.bmj.com/content/351/bmj.h4614.long.

Saletti-Cuesta L, Delgado A, Ortiz-Gomez T, Lopez-Fernandez LA. Diferencias de género en la percepción del logro profesional en especialistas de medicina familiar y comunitaria. *Rev. Esp. Salud Publica.* 2013; 87(3): 221-238. http://scielo.isciii.es/scielo.php?pid=S1135-57272013000300002&script=sci_arttext.

Turabian JL. Cuadernos de Medicina de Familia y Comunitaria. Una introducción a los principios de Medicina de Familia. Madrid: Díaz de Santos. 1995. http://www.amazon.co.uk/Cuadernos-medicina-familia-y-comunitaria/dp/8479781920.

Chapter 3

# The Family Doctor as a Drinker of Chinese Tea

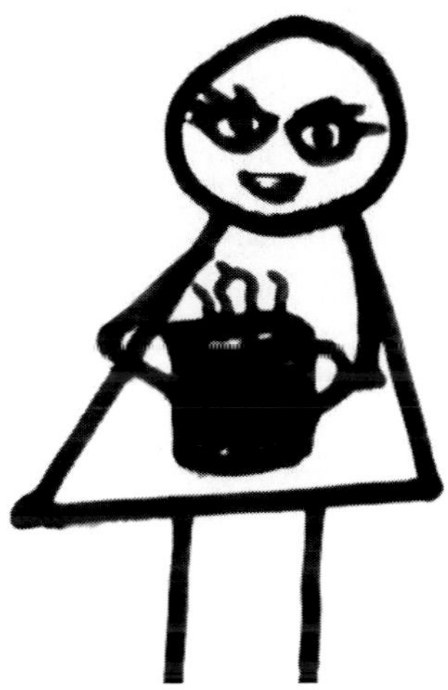

Every family doctor should have to read the *Book of Tea*. This is a very complete treatise on tea making that uses knowledge developed over two thousand years of tea preparation.

The poet, Lu Tong, of the dynasty Tang, said, "The first cup of tea wets the throat; the second removes the loneliness and melancholy; the third washes the intestines and helps to write books of 5 thousand characters; the fourth produced sweat that comes out through the pores taking the troubles; the fifth cleans the skin; the sixth makes us immortal and the seventh cannot be taken, because it would be like leaving the wind to pass through the two armpits."

Each day, the first patient that the family physician sees is like the first sip of tea, "happiness." The second patient of the day is "enjoyment," the third, "serenity," the fourth, "madness," and the fifth, "ecstasy"!

The family doctor does not need the snow water that falls onto the flowers of the plum tree because when this water falls onto the flowers it absorbs their perfume — which, according to Lu Wu is the best for making a good tea. It is sufficient for the inner harmony and desire of the family doctor to achieve "good" consultations: those that are useful for the patient and for him.

Thus, the first cup — the first patient seen every day — smokes on my lips and in my throat; the second patient violates my solitude; the third penetrates into my bowels and removes thousands of rare ideographs; the fourth patient bathes me in slight sweat and all the sorrows of my life are eliminated across my pores; with the fifth cup — the fifth patient — I am purified; the sixth transports me to the abode of the immortals. The seventh, ah, the seventh patient! But already you cannot drink any more. You can feel the breath of a cold aura inflating your sleeves. The family doctor, as a drinker of Chinese tea, has to take a break, and maybe has a cup of coffee! During this rest, perhaps the family doctor can say, as did the Chinese poet: "where is Horaisan, our paradise?" Ah! During this period of rest, perhaps the family doctor could say, as did the Chinese poet: "where is Horaisan, our paradise? Ah! Let me rise up on this sweet breeze, rock in its waves and let her lead me there."

## References

Fuxiang D y Mengliang L. El té chino. Beijing, República Popular China: Ediciones en Lenguas Extranjeras; 1990. p. 158.

Kerouac J. Los vagabundos del Dharma. Barcelona: Bruguera S.A.; 1981.

Lane K. The longest art. Exeter, Devon: The Royal College of General Practitioners; 1992.

McPhee J. Heirs of General Practice. New York: Farrar Straus Giroux; 1986.

Okakura K. El libro del té. Barcelona: Editorial Kairós; 1991.

*Chapter 4*

# The Family Doctor as an Optician

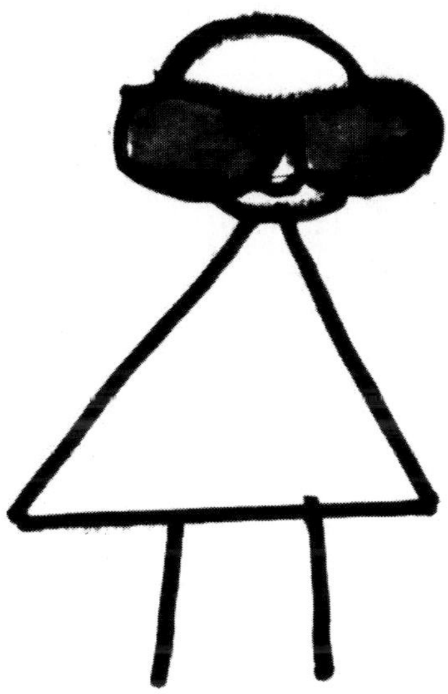

In 1927, the famous physicist, Neils Bohr, developed his theory of complementarity: trying to understand the nature of light, he discovered that light can be either a particle or a wave, and that this inconsistency occurs because it is not the light itself that we measure but the interactions with the light. Thus, we can show that light has the properties of a wave or a particle depending on the particular experiment we choose. In other words, this depends on our methodology.

The family doctor has to be an optician, choosing the correct "glasses" to be able to see the health problem. There are two main types of "glasses," the bio-psycho-social ones and the biomedical ones. Any glass distorts vision: through some glass the straight lines appear as curves and buildings, and walls are not straight but convex or slightly oval. With other glass the vision is also distorted: the curved lines appear as straight lines, and everything, including buildings and walls, appear to be straight. Thus, the world takes on a different form.

When we attend a patient, we see his problem in different forms according to our "glasses." Thus, we could have attended to a man who was presenting with a heart attack in a hospital emergency room. While he was there, there were many difficulties to take him a venous route, and several attempts failed. In the meantime, he went into cardiac arrest. We might exclaim: "How lucky had this patient to be in the emergency room 30 minutes before the arrest, thanks to this his life could be saved!"

But, shortly afterward we attend to another case, with other "glasses." This was another man who had a heart attack and was being treated in the hospital emergency room. While he was there, there were many difficulties to take him a venous route, and several attempts failed. In the meantime, he went into cardiac arrest. "Does the patient had had cardiac arrest if he had not been in the emergency room and go through the stressful experience?", the doctor wondered. "It is obvious that this patient's problems are located in systems outside of the heart," thought the doctor. "But, how strange it is! It is the same case! But through some glasses I see an organic cardiac problem, and through others a bio-psycho-social problem."

The majority of the doctors wear a specific pair of glasses. Once it is accepted that the problem is biomedical or psycho-social, the doctor adjusts his conduct and reactions in such a way that they fit with what he believes. When looking through these glasses, behaviour is adapting according to perception and it "proves our perception" and, as a consequence, it reinforces the perception.

These glasses are the theoretical framework for understanding what we see. The glasses — theoretical frameworks — are constructed with a predetermined ideology, history, and production time.

Family doctors should always wear two pairs of glasses to enable them see more and to avoid be locked into a single vision of reality. In this way, we will avoid seeing what "we want to see."

## References

Bucay J. Recuentos para Demián. México: Océano exprés; 2010.

Bui TC, Krieger HA, Blumenthal-Barby JS. Framing effects on physicians' judgment and decision making. *Psychol Rep.* 2015; 117(2):508-22. http://www.ncbi.nlm.nih.gov/pubmed/26444837.

http://www.amazon.co.uk/Cuadernos-medicina-familia-y-comunitaria/dp/8479781920.

Martorell JL. El guión de vida. Bilbao: Desclée De brouwer; 2000.

Perez Franco B, Turabian Fernandez JL. Framework of Competences of Family Doctors: Clinics or People? Aten Primaria 2007;39(1):41-3. http://www.elsevier.es/es-revista-atencion-primaria-27-articulo-marco-competencial-los-medicos-familia-13098264.

Turabian JL. Cuadernos de Medicina de Familia y Comunitaria. Una introducción a los principios de Medicina de Familia. Madrid: Díaz de Santos; 1995.

*Chapter 5*

# The Family Doctor as a Football Coach

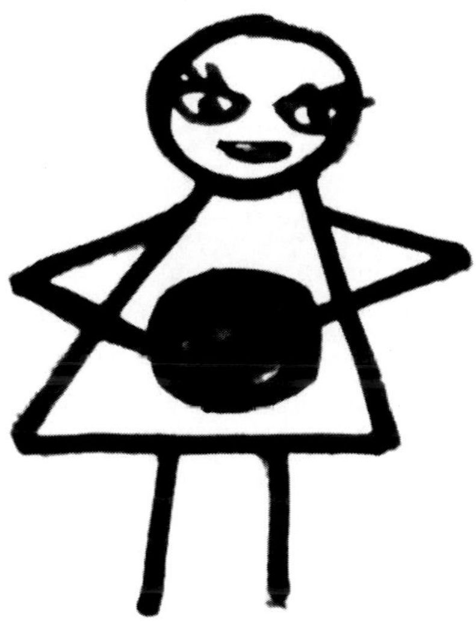

Many patients attended by the family doctor, seek "to be trained," to find a doctor who will guide them to improve. And here we have to consider the lessons of football coaches.

There are some lessons that the football coaches can offer to family doctors.

First: you can never say, "this player (patient) will not become famous."

Second: you can never say, "this player will become famous" (the stars of football admit that they had companions who were playing better than them, but for the lack of luck or because of a lack of interest they did not become famous).

Third: the coach almost always knows more than the pupil. There are patients who "play" in a particular position, but the coach can tell them: "look, you are a good patient, but if you want to improve, you have to learn to defend yourself"; this can be essential to achieving improvements and cures.

Fourth: never ignore his skill to dodge. The coach/family doctor focuses on how the player moves without the ball: when he is not a patient, when he accompanies a relative, or for the comments of these, or for their role in the family —his role as a resource.

Fifth: you must attack the will of your opponents, your teammates, and your coach. The player/patient must have individualism — catching the ball and start an impossible run towards the opposing goal — to raise their level and become the best.

Sixth (the most important): which the same patient provides!

In the same way that a coach manages the talent of the players without being the protagonist, family physicians as coaches of the patients can act to empower them to take advantage of their, often unexplored, qualities. The family doctor as coach controls the development of change, delegates to the players and manages their talents, encouraging them to achieve the maximum results that their situation will allow.

The trainer, as family doctor, works predominantly with adults and must therefore take into account the characteristics inherent in the concept of adult education, the sense of perspective that allows us to establish judgements about ourselves and about others, as well as being responsible for oneself. These results in a sense of complete development or personal growth, the utilization of individual talents (maturity), and the sense of autonomy gained from a voluntary decision-making capacity.

## References

Blanchard K, Shula D. Everyone' s a coach. Five business secrets for high-performance coaching. New York: Harper Business; 1995.

Christina RW, Corcos DM. Coaches guide to teaching sport skills. Champaign, Illinois: Human Kinetics; 1988.

Cook. Soccer coaching. The professional way. London: A & C Black Publishers Ltd.; 2006.

Cooper HN, Goldman KD, Schmalz KJ. Got Game? The Role of Coaches and Coaching in Improving Your Career and Life "Games." Health Promot Pract 2013;14 801-804. http://hpp.sagepub.com/cgi/content/full/14/6/801?etoc.

Earley PC, Erez M. The transplanted executive. Oxford: Oxford University Press; 1997.

Editorial. Joys of (top-notch) supervision. *Nature.* 2005; 434(421). http://www.nature.com/nature/journal/v434/n7032/full/434421a.html.

Murray M, Owen MA. Beyond the myths and magic of mentoring. How to facilitate an effective mentoring program. San Francisco: Jossey-Bass Publishers; 1991.

Parsole E. Coaching, mentoring and assessing. A practical guide to developing competence. London: Kogan Page; 1995.

Rogers A. Teaching adults. Buckingham: Open University Press; 1996.

Senge P. La Quinta Disciplina. Barcelona: Granica; 1992.

Stevens N. *Learn to coach*. Oxford: How To Book Ltd.; 2005.

*Chapter 6*

# The Family Doctor as a Cathedral Builder

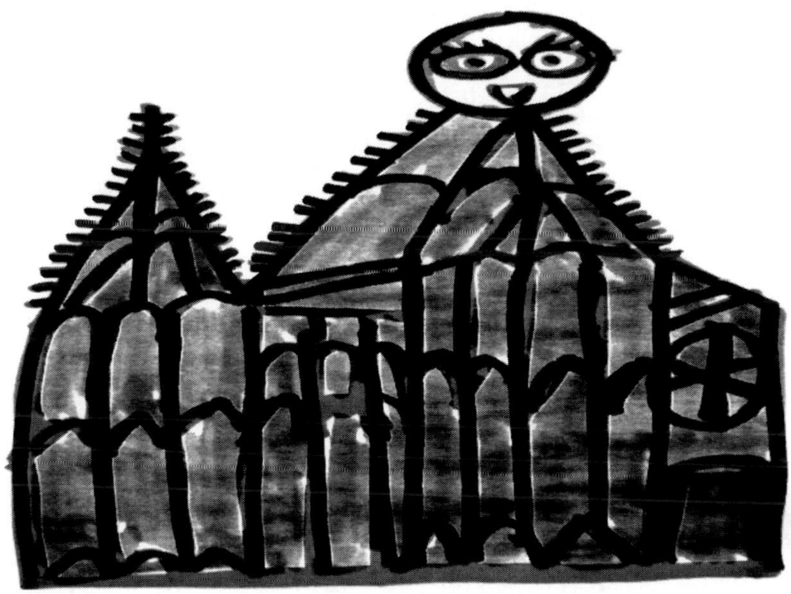

The family doctor as the builder of Gothic cathedrals re-uses the stones of the previous building, introducing them into the foundations of the new one. In so doing, he uses all the personal and familiar precedents. He does not neglect anything, and the earlier periods join with the most recent expression. The family doctors and the cathedrals builders journey from the visible manifestation in the current moment back to the initial principles, from the embouchure to the sources.

The family doctor as the builder of Gothic cathedrals has to learn from the material, the techniques and the history; he has to have a sensibility to Nature. He has to communicate so that the individuals understand and complete each other with the intention of constituting a coherent society. He also needs to perceive the mysteries of the life, using instruments of reflection about the Universe and about oneself that unite reason and intuition. As Saint

Augustine said, "The most important thing is to meditate on the meaning of a fact and not to discuss its authenticity."

As in the construction of a cathedral, in the care of each patient the family doctor must achieve a proportion or harmony between the parts and the whole, a "sense of the essential." The family doctor tries to achieve a kind of knowledge as slender as an outrigger, as powerful as a tower, as serene as an apse.

Under the influence of positivism, the modern world believed that reason can explain everything. In contrast, the Middle Ages unreservedly supported the unknown and did not try to force it into the framework of logic. In the quarry of the cathedral, as in the consultation room of family medicine, there is a mystery, a mystery whose substance a young apprentice can perceive without being able to explain it himself.

The family doctor, as the builder cathedrals, works with symbols. In the Middle Ages, facts were translated into symbols. The symbol is a sign that leads to knowledge that is impossible to find through any other form. The symbol is a way of moving from one plane to another, from matter to spirit.

To Gothic cathedral represents the union between the sky and the land. The cathedrals appear to us as places where each of the elements of the building seeks to infuse people with consciousness of the greatness of the divine. The family doctor appears as the professional who seeks to join body and mind.

The technical elements of the cathedrals fundamentally identify advances in Gothic architecture. Two elements that appear as the basis of Gothic architecture in general are the pointed arch and the groin vault. With the use of the pointed arch the highest elevation of the building is achieved, thus contributing to reinforcing the upward direction of the cathedral. The vaulted walls lighten the walls, obtaining a joint that provides a major elevation and lighting to the temple.

The technical contributions of the family doctor, such as the gothic cathedral, are the person-centered approach ("elevation"), and the contextualization of the patient — family, labour, and community (the system of buttresses that secures the building to the ground).

## References

Cassell E. *The Nature of Suffering and the Goals of Medicine.* Oxford: Oxford University Press; 1991.

Jacq C, Brunier F. El mensaje de los constructores de catedrales. Barcelona: Plaza y Janes, S.A.; 1976.

Piquero López MAB. Las catedrales góticas castellanas. Salamanca: Ediciones Colegio de España, 1992.

*Chapter 7*

# The Family Doctor as a Potato in the Basement

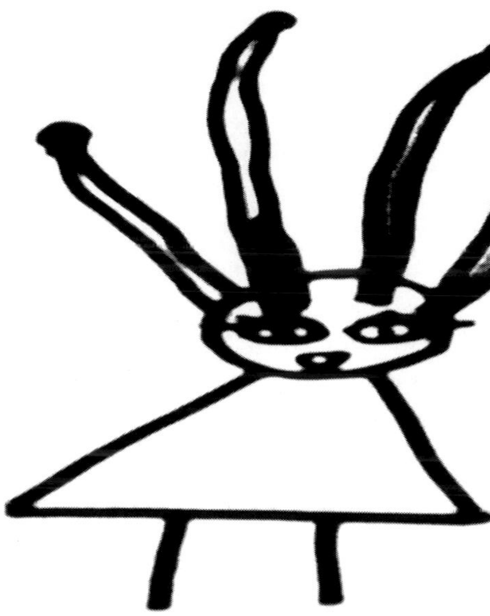

The family doctor must have a specific or innate skill for growth and development regardless of the conditions he might face.

C. Rogers calls this innate force of development the "tendency to upgrade," and tells a story of his childhood to describe its meaning. "I remember in my childhood the potatoes which we keep in the winter as a reserve were in the basement, several meters below a small cellar window. The conditions were unfavourable, but the potatoes came to have white and pale outbreaks and these weak outbreaks could grow 1 to 2 meters in height and reach the light of the window," In spite of the problems that hindered their growth, the potatoes (and all organisms) show that they can develop. Each organism, including humans, has this ability to make the most of its context.

The family doctor must have this ability to grow himself, and to help his patients to grow. The core of the interview between the family doctor and his patient is this belief that everything can grow. This belief means that the family doctor trusts in his skill to make the correct choices for his way of life. The family doctor encourages this development by promoting the necessary conditions for a healthy growth. There are three crucial conditions that the family doctor offers the patient to create a therapeutic context:

- Empathy
- Acceptance (positive and unconditional)
- Congruence.

Each individual has the natural ability to grow and to personally develop — to change and grow emotionally in a way that is appropriate to each person. Personal development involves:

- A great self-awareness (learning about who we are and how we think, feel and act)
- An appropriate set of values, beliefs and attitudes (what we really value and what is important in our lives)
- What we want to obtain (our goals and ambitions).

## References

Buchanan L, Hughes R. Experiences of person-centred counselling training. A compendium of case studies to assist prospective applicants. Herefordshire: PCCS Books; 2000.
Cortese A. El libro de la buena suerte:(Buenos Aires: Mega Libros, 1998.
De Bono E. Future Positive. London: Penguin Books; 1979.
Rain Man. Wikipedia. [homepage on the Internet]. https://en.wikipedia.org/wiki/Rain_Man.
Rogers CR. A way of being. New York: Houghton Mifflin Company; 1995.
Rogers CR. Client-centered therapy. London: Constable; 1998.
Tounier P. The Healing of Persons. London: Collins; 1966.

*Chapter 8*

# The Family Doctor as a Jazz Musician

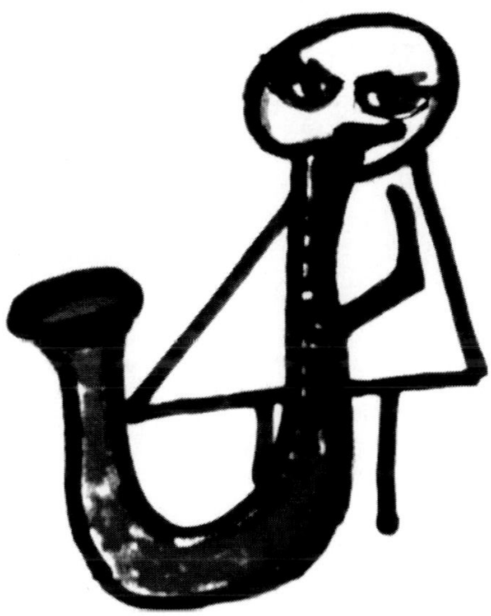

The improvisation of a jazz musician in one piece, within an overall musical structure, gives the sense of collective creation and interdependent responsibility.

The trumpeter in a jazz band is one of the musicians and he is not external to them. He does not perform from the front, but as one member of the set. He provides a great freedom of musical expression to the components of the band and facilitates their individual and collective splendour. He determines the parts of the repertoire and beats time. He is creative, funny. His facilitative leadership channels energies, and he is one more member of the team.

The music that the "family doctor plays in each office is a music that sounds like jazz: it has great variability, contexts, patterns, models, actors and relationships with potential interactions." Everyone is different, and therefore his families, his environments, his expectations, his problems, his desires, are also different.

The traditional view that the best way to improve health care is to eliminate the variability is not held in family medicine —a complex adaptive system — whose actors (patients, families, contexts, and doctors, health systems, context) interact in a nonlinear way.

Here, the health care is a response to changing circumstances, as is the case in the improvisation of the jazz musician.

The interview between the doctor and the patient goes beyond the structured protocols, and, in a search for our own style, we must "pass through them" to understand the patient and ourselves. The good jazz musician has his own speech since, through his technical skills he has learned to know and to play his best "notes." Above all, he is a good musician because he listens to other musicians and has learned to improvise his "musical" answers, focusing on understanding and feeling each musical phrase without a predefined guide.

Therefore, the family doctor should be a jazz musician.

## References

Haidet P. Jazz and the 'Art' of Medicine: Improvisation in the Medical Encounter. *Ann Fam Med.* 2007; 5:164-169. http://www.annfammed.org/cgi/content/full/5/2/164.

Miller WL, Reuben R. McDaniel, Jr, Crabtree BF, Stange KC. Practice Jazz: Understanding Variation in Family Practices Using Complexity Science. *J Fam Pract.* 2001;50(10):872-878. http://www.jfponline.com/index.php?id=22143&tx_ttnews[tt_news]=168286.

Reid S. Music as a metaphor for the medical consultation. South African Family Practice. 2008; 50 (1): 62-64. http://dx.doi.org/10.1080/20786204.2008.10873670.

*Chapter 9*

# The Family Doctor as a Knife with Multiple Uses (Swiss Army Knife)

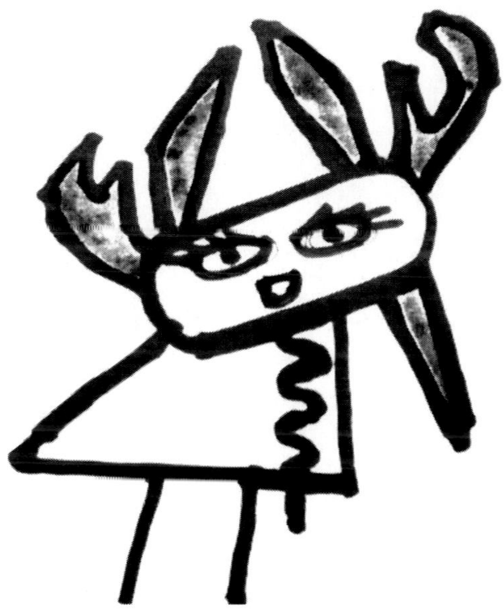

This image highlights the huge number of tools available to a knife or razor, such as the Swiss army knife, and the different uses that can be given to each of them. The availability of this "great little resort" helps you out of virtually any trouble. Besides, being manufactured in Switzerland it is of high quality and uses sophisticated technology.

The doctor of the future will not be the super specialist in a very small plot, but will have the ability to adapt to any challenge. This will involve a transformation of professional profiles for many medical specialties. The family doctor has a role as a facilitator-leader. The family physician is a multipurpose, multi-resource, and eminently practical person: a simple box with powerful tools that are available to any professional of primary care. This is what is called having the profile of a Swiss army knife: a professional who is able to adapt to any context.

Accepting these characteristics as desirable is a critique of the current university model, a requires a move from a closed program (in which the content is imposed) to an open design that allows the apprentice to learn what s/he want, and one that understands and thinks about their training needs according to the changing contexts. We must be prepared to face this challenge and students need to be proactive, the curricula of future family doctors should have the profile of a Swiss army knife.

## References

Bowman MA. TOP Docs: Family Physicians with Competing Demands and the Right Priorities—Individual, Family, and Community Health. *J Am Board Fam Med.* 2009; 22(2): 110-112. http://www.jabfm.org/content/22/2/110.full.

Brewster B, Mills J. The Doctor. *Just another year*. London: BBC Books; 1991.

How the work of family doctors has changed. BBC News. Health. 16 November 2013. http://www.bbc.com/news/health-24955762.

http://www.amazon.es/Actividades-comunitarias-medicina-atenci%C3%B3n-primaria/dp/8479784741.

Inteligencias múltiples. Los siete estilos de aprendizaje. Monografías. Com. 14 de febrero de 2003. http://www.monografias.com/cgi-bin/jump.cgi?ID=38465.

Turabian JL, Pérez Franco B. Actividades Comunitarias en Medicina de Familia y Atención Primaria. Madrid: Díaz de Santos; 2001.

Winckler M. La enfermedad de Sachs. Madrid: Ediciones Akal S.A.; 1999.

Chapter 10

# The Family Doctor as a Myopic Hawk

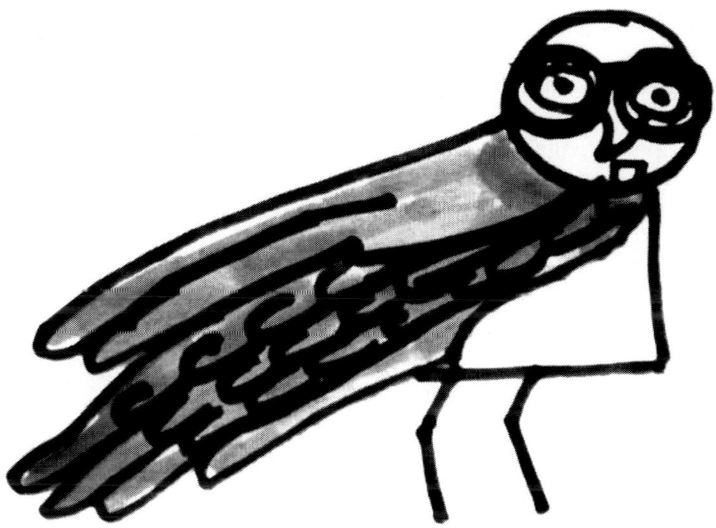

We can distinguish two basic processes in thinking: the broad or general approach and that which is specific or detailed.

Imagine two falcons. One has great eyesight but the other is short-sighted. Both feed on frogs, mice and lizards. The hawk with good eyesight can recognize a frog from a great height and eats. Since this hawk has such good eyesight it can live on frogs and soon forgets about mice and lizards. The hawk that does not have good eyesight cannot do the same. This hawk needs to create a general concept of "small moving things." Whenever he sees something small moving he flies down to catch it. Sometimes he gets a frog, a mouse or a lizard and, occasionally, a child's toy.

Although the hawk with good eyesight might initially be considered to be superior, this depends on what aspects are considered. If the frogs disappear, the hawk with good eyesight would die, whereas the myopic hawk would continue to live with few alterations to his way of life. This is because the myopic hawk has the flexibility that comes from the rather large and fuzzy concept of "small things moving."

The human brain does not immediately form accurate and detailed images but works from general, broad, and vague views, which go on to become concepts. These broad, general, and vague images are extremely useful for thought. Good thinkers have the ability to avoid getting stuck in the detail, they know how to generalize, and from there they return to the specific and the general. Good family physicians also have that ability. When seeking a solution to a problem we first look at it in very broad terms. These broad and vague concepts allow us to look more widely and flexibly, and to evaluate options.

## References

De Bono E. Aprende a pensar por ti mismo. Barcelona: Paidós; 1977.

Fry J. Common Diseases. Their Nature, Incidence and Care. Lancaster, England: MTP Press Ltd;1987.

Gómez Ocaña JM, Revilla Pascual E, Fernández-Cuesta Valcarce MA, El-Asmar Osman A. Las 50 principales consultas en medicina de familia. Agencia Laín Entralgo. Salud Madrid. Comunidad de Madrid. Madrid: CEGE Taller Editorial; 2011.

Hart JT. A new Kind of Doctor. The General Practitioner's Part In the Health of Community. London: Merlin Press; 1988.

*Chapter 11*

# The Family Doctor as a Classic Painter

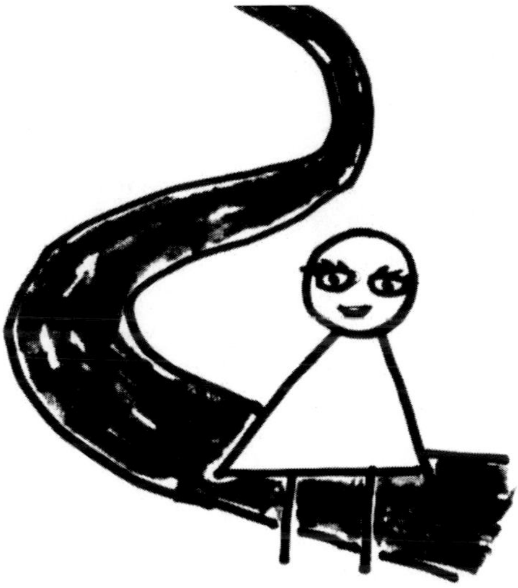

The bio-psychosocial elements of diseases have been described as long-term "paths." The family doctor also acquires a visual or mental trajectory from the presentation of symptoms at each patient's visit.

In movies or in classic paintings there are certain sequences that introduce visual motion diagrams as "paths of sight." These refer to a specific order of representation in which the artist wants to describe certain events arranged along a path. In addition, there is usually something in the painting that attracts our attention prior to all other elements. From this point, the artist moves the focus along the desired path. This trajectory can be described as a line of movement, with a trail of graduated tints or groupings or "game" characters. In different works of plastic art this "line" — the course of movement or the trajectory — can be traced ways other than the purely linear. For example, the can be achieved by changing hues within the structure of light images or colour, or by the successive splitting of volumes and distances.

In the doctor-patient relationship during the clinical interview, the communication is pointing and guiding our path of sight. Many clinical presentations begin, not with a physical diagnosis, but with a point that attracts our attention and usually involves psychosocial issues relevant to both the patient and the doctor. This is similar to looking at frames in the sequence of a film (for example, the scene of the battle on the frozen lake in the film *Alexander Nevsky*, by Eisenstein, where we find a correspondence between the movement of the music and the movement of the eye on the artistic composition). This is also present when we look at a classic painting. For example, in, *The meeting between San Antonio and San Pablo*, painted by Sassetta, the "trajectory of sight" is linked to a way forward rather than back through the paint. Similarly, during the doctor-patient interview, the eye of family doctor is focuses on certain places narrated by the patient.

This can be seen in the painting of the *Adoration of the Magi* by Gentile da Fabriano (1423, Uffizi Gallery, Florence). This composition lacks geometric structure and it must be "read" as a text or a story, starting at the upper left corner where the Three Magi who are near the sea and discover the star that will guide them. Following the path between the gentle slopes and the farmlands, we see them as they enter Jerusalem under the central arch. In the left window is their departure. The central field becomes the direction of travel, which is directed towards us. Suddenly, from a deep ravine surrounded by a rocky wall and a hedge, comes a human tide. We can already make out every detail of the faces, dresses, weapons, and the horses' harnesses. The luxurious train of cavalry and infantry, and in which we also see hunters, race-horses, and exotic animals, halts when they reach their goal. Just then, the young king, who appears in the foreground whilst a page is taking away his spurs, kneels and prepares to deliver his offering.

## References

Eorsi A. La pintura gótica internacional. Título original: Az internacionális gótika festészete. Budapest: Corvina Klado; 1984. La Habana: Editorial Arte y Literatura; 1984.

Freud S. Psicoanálisis del arte. Madrid: Alianza Editorial; 1978.

http://www.elsevier.es/es/revistas/semergen-medicina-general--familia-40/como-abrir-puerta-comprension-los-sintomas-medicina-90055375-formacion-continuada-2011.

http://www.elsevier.es/es-revista-atencion-primaria-27-articulo-senderos-clinicos-presentacion-los-sintomas-90151784.

Knox JDE. Presentations in primary care. London: Bitterworths;1985.

Siebeck R. Medicina en movimiento. Barcelona: Editorial Científico-Médica; 1957.

Stewart M, Brown JB, Weston WW, McWhinney IR, McWilliam CL, Freeman TR. Patient-centered medicine. Transforming the clinical method. London: SAGE Publications; 1995.

Turabian Jl, Pérez Franco B. Clinical pathways in the presentation of symptoms. considered as a plastic work of art in Family Medicine. Aten Primaria. 2012;44:511-3.

Turabián JL, Pérez Franco B. How is the door of understanding of the symptoms opened in family medicine? SEMERGEN. 2011; 37 (10):554.

Turabián JL, Pérez Franco B. The symptoms in family medicine are not symptoms of disease. they are symptoms of life. Aten Primaria 2012;44(4):232-236. http://www.elsevier.es/es/revistas/atencion-primaria-27/los-sintomas-medicina-familia-no-son-sintomas-90119927-articulo-especial-2012.

*Chapter 12*

# The Family Doctor as an Explorer on a Desert Island

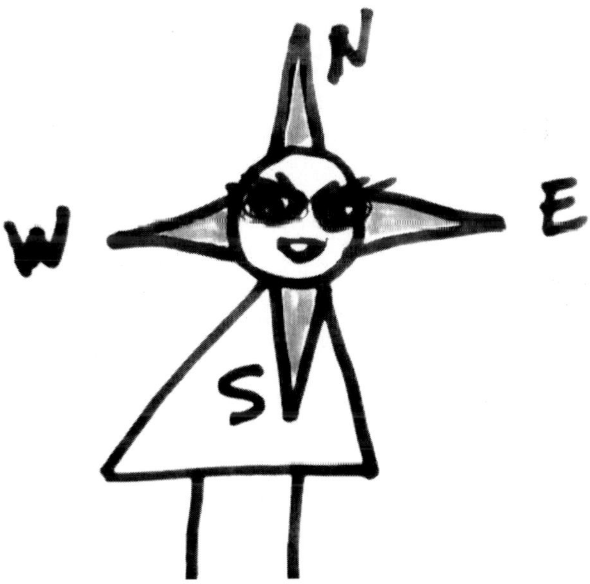


One ability of the family doctor must be to know how to "draw attention," that is, how to make an observation or systematic reflection. The questions the doctor asks are resources for directing attention.

When an explorer returns from an expedition to a newly discovered island he tells of a smoking volcano and a bird that could not fly. But what else was there? He noted that those were the two things that caught his attention. That is not enough. And so he is sent back to the island with specific instructions to use a very simple method for directing his attention. "Look to the north and record what you see. Then look south and note what you see. Then look east and note what you see. Then west and record what you see. Now come back and give us your scrapbook." This N-S-E-W instruction provides a simple method for directing our attention.

Our attention generally flows in three ways:

1. What captures our interest or involves us emotionally at the time.
2. Care habits established through experience and practice.
3. A more or less random change of course from one place to another.

The family doctor has to deliberately direct your attention to N-S-E-W, not to lose any important aspect of patient.

## References

De Bono E. Aprende a pensar por ti mismo. Barcelona: Paidós; 1977.

Defoe D. Aventuras de Robinson Crusoe. Estella, Navarra: Salvat Editores, S.A.; 1983.

Morgan WL, Engel G.L. The clinical approach to the patient. London: W. B. Saunders Company; 1969.

Turabián JL, Pérez Franco B. The diagnostic concept in family medicine: A view of the landscape. The diagnosis in family medicine. Aten Primaria. 2010;42(2):66-69. http://www.elsevier.es/es-revista-atencion-primaria-27-articulo-el-concepto-diagnostico-medicina-familia-ver-un-13146911.

*Chapter 13*

# The Family Doctor as a Bass

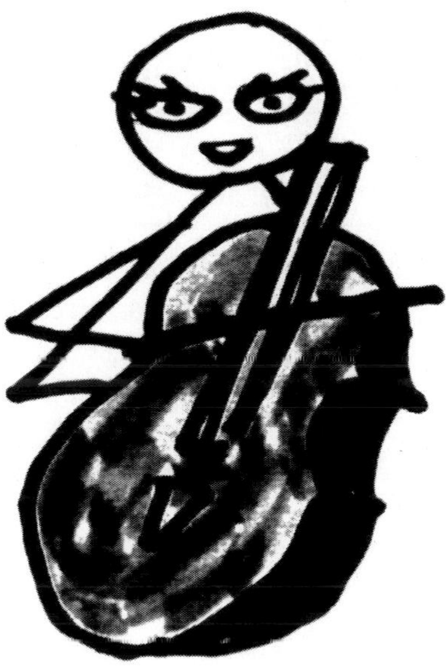

The bass and basso continuo is a metaphor that explains the basis of the work of the family doctor.

Each task of the diagnostic and therapeutic process is a musical bass that has to harmonize all the data and contextual the microcosm of the patient, facing the uncertainty generated by the symphony of multi-morbidity and poly-pharmacy. The effort to make the bass sound is similar to the methodology necessary to develop reflection and dialogue in the work of the family doctor: it is hardly perceptible but it is irreplaceable.

The health system within which the family doctor works not only tries to reduce disease, but also seeks to affirm the individual and people's social development. The bass helps to build the apacity to meet the various forms of health problems, to achieve the skills of medical practice, and methodological and didactic action: its inter-textuality or dialogue of ideas deals with the conflicts and uncertainties associated with the management of knowledge.

The family doctor's tasks of diagnosis and treatment should have a "basso continuo" that must be present throughout his work. In the Baroque and Renaissance (when polyphony existed) there was no conductor to lead a group of musicians. Instead they used what is now known as "continuo," to mark the rhythm that guided the instruments. The continuo is an accompaniment technique. The continuo is executed by one or several instruments: typically a harmonic instrument (i.e., one that is able to produce chords or polyphony), as keyboard instruments (harpsichord, organ), and others such as the harp and the lute, plus, simultaneously an instrument such as a cello, bassoon, or bass.

The "basso continuo" of the family doctor, which allows for improvisation and personal touch, is a technique for accompanying the patient throughout the diagnostic process and is the place where other diagnostic instruments improvise.

## References

http://apps.elsevier.es/watermark/ctl_servlet?_f=10&pident_articulo=90443461&pident_usuario=0&pcontactid=&pident_revista=27&ty=22&accion=L&origen=zonadelectura&web=www.elsevier.es&lan=es&fichero=27v47n09a90443461pdf001.pdf.

Jaulin Plana C. El contrabajo: análisis de las organizaciones. Hergue Editora Andaluza; 2008.

Kandinsky. De lo espiritual en el arte. Barcelona: Barral Editores, S. A.; 1982.

Turabián JL, Samarín-Ocampo E, Minier L, Pérez-Franco B. Learning concepts of diagnosis in family medicine: the ''mark Robinson sign'' – the traces that should not be there. Aten Primaria. 2015; 47(9): 596-602. http://www.elsevier.es/ct-revista-atencion-primaria-27-articulo-aprendiendo-conceptos-del-diagnostico-medicina-90443461.

*Chapter 14*

# The Family Doctor as a Plug

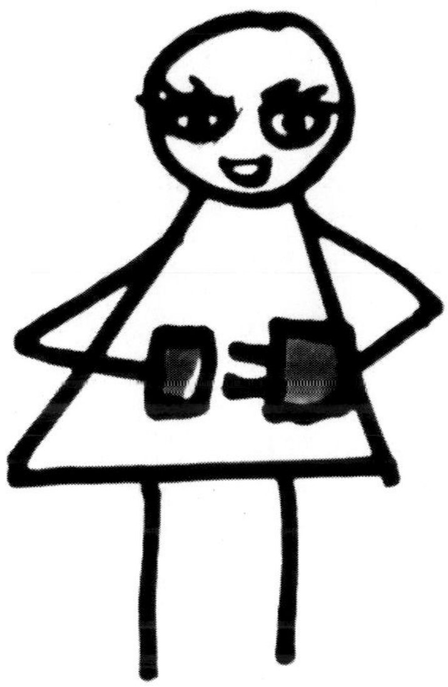

The term “plug” is used here as a verb that means connecting a device to the network. This is an action of great importance to the family doctor.

From a holistic point of view the concepts of sickness and health, "be alive" means "be related" and "be related" means build those relationships. Being healthy is not something that is fixed or that people are “locked” into, it is possible see changes and alternatives. The evolution, change, learning, healing, and adaptation of a living organism (a person, a patient) always depend on the individual and the surrounding context. Being sick is to be “locked” in a black tunnel without end, not knowing what to do to improve things. Degradation (disease, aging) that occurs over time in a living system is primarily the result of a breakdown or reduction of interconnections or relationships.

Therefore, be “locked off” because the connection has failed (the system or context) [as in a computer], is the concept of “being sick” to the family doctor. And thus the healing (treatment, intervention of the family doctor) becomes possible through its participation in the matrix of communication with others, “reconnecting” the patient with the matrix of relationships. To the family doctor healing, in one way or another, means returning the part to the whole. You have to "take the electric cables and plug them in again."

The traumatic overflow entailed in sickness may also lead to a fragmented connection with oneself through various forms of dissociation such as panic, silence, isolation, blockage, exaggerated manifestations or temporal and spatial disorientation. The interruption of the connections can be both the cause and the result of overflowing life experiences. A traumatized person who is disconnected from themselves and disoriented in time and space, is not fully able to positively connect with others, including their partner, their family of origin, and their cultural and spiritual roots. Therefore, in the same way that an individual may feel overwhelmed and be traumatized, it is important to remember that this phenomenon can also be applied to entire families.

In essence, the concept of "disease" has to do with the fact of being overwhelmed and with dropped connections. The circumstances and events that can overwhelm one person might be manageable for another person. There are, of course, experiences that would overwhelm anyone. Trauma may result from a sudden shock and also a series of difficult and painful experiences that accumulate over time. In the latter case, a seemingly minimal event can cause a post-traumatic response that actually stems from previous events, consciously or not remembered.

As a good "plug" the family doctor must understand that efforts that focus only on the somatic to restore balance within these biological systems are not sufficient to explain, resolve or break these patterns of disease, which can also reappear at a later in time. The family physician as a plug has to understand that traumatic events occur in a wider context than might be assumed from a linear perspective or from one context alone. As Nietzsche suggested, "every time we doubt our right to have its own mission and start doing an easy task, whatever, the result is always the disease."

## References

http://www.elsevier.es/es/revistas/atencion-primaria-27/mas-farmacos-curar-las-alteraciones-las-relaciones-13083930-cartas-al-director-2006.

Koven S. The Doctor's New Dilemma. *N Engl J Med* 2016; 374:608-609. http://www.nejm.org/doi/full/10.1056/NEJMp1513708.

Nietzsche F. Verdad y mentira en sentido extramoral. Miscelánea de opiniones y sentencias. Madrid: Grupo Editorial Marte, S.A.; 1988.

Shem S. Monte Miseria. Barcelona: Anagrama, 2000.

St. Just A. Un patrón fractal en el tiempo. Equilibrio Relativo en un Mundo Inestable: Una investigación sobre Educación de Traumas y Recuperación. Buenos Aires: Alma Lepik; 2007.

Turabián Fernández JL, Pérez Franco B. Notes on "resolutivity" and "cure" in family medicine. *Aten Primaria.* 2003; 32:296-9. http://www.elsevier.es/es-revista-atencion-primaria-27-articulo-apuntes-resolutividad-cura-medicina-familia-13051598.

Turabián-Fernández JL, Pérez-Franco. More Drugs to Cure Disorders in Human Relations? The Case of Addiction to Tobacco. *Aten Primaria* 2006;37(1):62-63.

*Chapter 15*

# The Family Doctor as a Musician

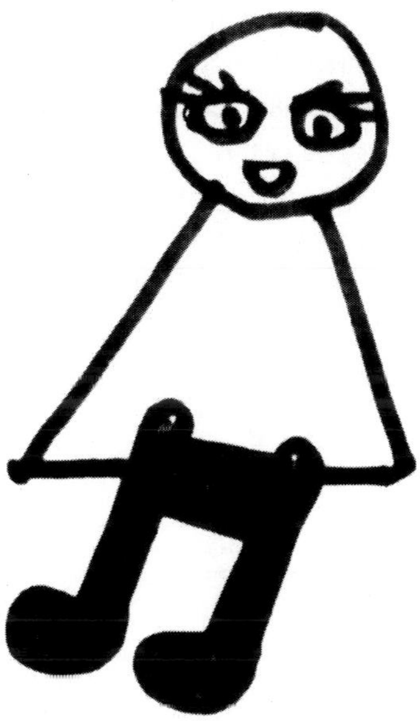

The relationship between doctor and patient resembles the act of playing music: a musician spends much of his time tuning the instrument, and also to practicing.

For the family doctor, the medical instrument is himself. The same doctor is the drug; when the doctor ordering tests, these depends on the physician attitudes toward risk and own personal factors; diagnostic errors can be attributed to the doctor's feelings about the patient; the background of the doctor and his family greatly influence the way in which he practices medicine (career choice, role in the family, myths, culture, and so on); the responses of the doctor to the problems of his own life and family, affect solutions professional problems.

At each consultation visit the family doctor should compare the patient with the mental images he has created over the years of life: from his experience as a child, a medical student, perhaps a father (that give rise to a conception of organic and psychological health), with what he learned in his study of histology, pathology and bacteriology. At each patient, the family doctor compares his internal person with patient. The patient also follows this same process. However, both people can work together: making music, and making an emotional experience possible.

If this "musical" potential is avoided, the doctor-patient relationship becomes a mechanical or commercial transaction: the patient is considered as a machine that is studied by another machine. The following methods are valid for helping the physician to become more conscious of their strength in the consultation: reflection, psychotherapy, case review, video of consultations, group approaches (Balint groups), groups of staff awareness, etc., and the playing of music!

## References

Balint E, Norell JS (Editors). Six minutes for the patient: interactions in general practice consultations. London: Tavistock publications; 1973.

Balint M, Hunt J, Joyce D, Marinker M, Woodcock J. Treatment or diagnosis. A study of repeat prescriptions in general practice. London: Tavistock Publications; 1984.

Lustig M. Balint groups: an Australasian perspective for psychiatrists. Australas Psychiatry. 2016; 24(1): 30-33. http://apy.sagepub.com/content/24/1/30?etoc.

McKensey. Balint groups – helping trainee psychiatrists make even better use of themselves Australas Psychiatry. 2016; 24(1): 84-87. http://apy.sagepub.com/content/24/1/84?etoc.

Moreau A. Formation psychologique en médecine et groupe balint. Beauvechain (Belgique): Nauwelaerts Editions; 1990.

*Chapter 16*

# The Family Doctor as an Adventurer

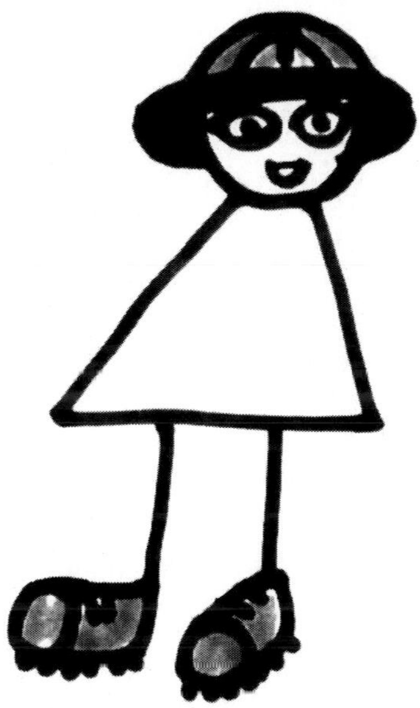

The family doctor is like a traveller journeying through unknown, unexplored places which we know almost nothing about, maybe the jungle; breaking through with lush greenery with a machete, or sailing, sometimes rapidly and sometimes slowly, along a mysterious river which, at times, has vast stretches of water whose banks are leagues apart, and at others are narrow channels.

The family doctor encounters unknown "adventures" within the first 10 minutes of each consultation and must colonize uncharted territories. He has to be traveller, a wanderer, restless, fearless and curious.

The family physician uses the clinical interview with the patient as a means of communication where the doctor-patient relationship occurs and develops. And it is this communication in the doctor-patient relationship that signals a forest trail or smoke from a fire in the jungle that helps us to focus our field study on the natural values of the place, or to wade through a desert or river, or to cross a valley — the clinical setting.

The family doctor needs good knowledge of "survival tactics in the wild" because when the family doctor attends to a patient, there may be a series of events that a pioneer and adventurer of the unknown must cope with confidently. The patient raises a problem; it's like coming to a river. The family doctor sees shining water and is located on the banks of a river that offers a waterway to the sea. What happens to the patient? Does the patient have hypertension, diabetes, depression, flu? Should the case go to review? What controls and procedures are adequate for follow up?

The family doctor begins a journey through the mountains. He has already made this journey but the road today he does not know well. A mountain blocks his passage. When he reached the top ledge it was so narrow that the stones were rolling before him. The landscape was mountain after mountains separated by green valleys. Who is this patient and where he is? What are the background, context and patient-family-physician relationship? What does the genogram tell us? The family doctor is in danger! He saw people approaching through the woods. Who are they? His heart is pounding ... wild! And then, dark clouds begin to appear in the sky. Does the patient present a serious problem? Is this post-infarction heart failure?

This results in new setbacks and concerns for the family doctor. The gentle breeze that pushed him down the river has suddenly disappeared; the sun has darkened and all of heaven has taken on a deep yellow hue. Presents complications in his evolution the patient?

But the traveller continues to advance for that unknown and dangerous territory. Will there be more adventures for the family doctor in the jungle? Natural noise in those thick forests was scarce, but occasionally howling was heard in the background of the jungle. The observer is in a state of nervousness. Has he sensed something bad? Has the patient has an adverse reaction? Care must be taken in these adventures in the jungle. Along the way there is a great and horrible serpent, creeping toward him, looking haughty. Will there be drug interactions with the drugs taken by the patient?

The family doctor continues downstream and slides into the middle of the river where the current pushes the family doctor quickly, without having to use the oars. Has the patient developed any other complications? Does the family doctor change or adjust the prescription, for example, in case of kidney failure?

And the journey ends. Finally the family doctor reaches the safety of a bay, and with great joy sees the city spread out along the coast.

So, what is the most basic survival tactic in the wild? "When following a river always do it in the direction of the water."

# References

Darwin C. The Voyage of the Beagle. Ware, Hertfordshire: Wordworth editions Limited; 1997.

http://www.elsevier.es/es/revistas/atencion-primaria-27/el-efecto-ver-primera-vez-mar-un-13128570-reflexiones-medicina-familia-2008.

http://www.elsevier.es/es/revistas/atencion-primaria-27/mapas-aventura-13118069-cartas-al-director-2008.

Paul Theroux. El Tao del viajero. Madrid: Santillana Ediciones Generales, S. L.; 2011.

Schweitzer A. More from the Primaveral Forest. London: Collins. Fontana Books; 1958.

Schweitzer A. My Life and Thought. London. Guild Books; 1957.

Turabian Fernandez JL, Perez Franco B. Map Towards Adventure. *Aten Primaria* 2008;40(4):209-216.

Turabián JL, Pérez Franco B. El efecto de ver por primera vez el mar. Un intento de definición de la Ley General de la medicina de familia: la entrevista es la clínica. *Aten Primaria.* 2008;40(11):565-6.

Westwood J. Sacred Journeys, New York; Henry Holt and Company; 1997.

*Chapter 17*

# The Family Doctor as a Photographer

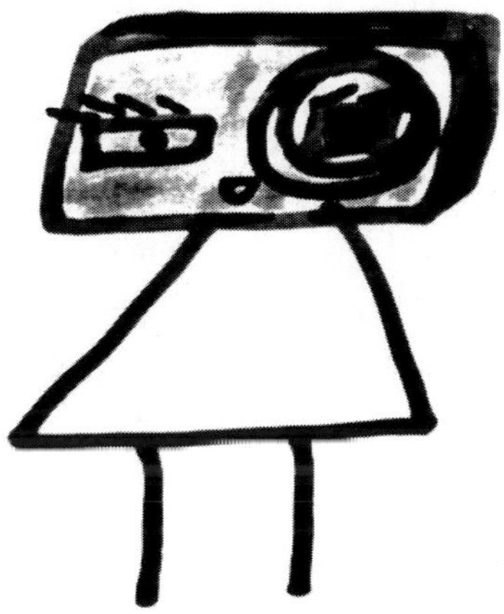

To change the “mental computer processing unit" of hospital care, “go to the border and, from there, look at the territory that you have left.”

The photograph is the territory to rcmcmbcr latcr.

The family doctor as photographer highlights the ability to observe and understand reality. A “panoramic” view provides a broader perspective for looking at the context, using a “zoom” lens he can see detail, and he has the freedom to “focus” on a topic of discussion or consultation in the smallest detail. The family doctor as a photographer is a curious, tireless, and adventurous seeker of “situations” and “perspectives” from which to understand reality.

The modus operandi of the family doctor as photographer is that who has a preference for unhappy and unpleasant places, or those aspects of human nature more brushed aside, or depicting the interiors of the rooms as the dining room and kitchen, showing an inner vision, with reflections of love and hate of the residents of those rooms.

This modus operandi is similar to family medicine in that it uses methods that are “dirty,” encounters sullen subjects, has casual meetings, uses therapeutic trials and anecdotal observations, and places faith in decisive moments. What contributes to the greater glory of family medicine is not innovation in the tool available and in efficiency (which we can leave to the manager, the bureaucrat, or the computer), but also in the depth of feeling. As family doctors we are involved in the relationships and the images that these provide us.

A tip for family doctor with less experience is to forget the diagnosis and treatment. A decision on diagnosis and treatment will occur, but family medicine is actually about relations and people management. It is about helping the sick through the borders of their fears and doubts and deep wounds, about managing the incalculable steps of the unexpected. Do not misunderstand. Family doctors are grateful to the tools that have given us clinical-knowledge, discipline, and drugs that sometimes work. But we must also recognize that the center of academic medicine is a monolith of truth and knowledge construction that simultaneously reveals a dark area influenced by unknown forces and powerful biases.

The achievements of family medicine are like the photos of certain photographers — often not totally clear or nice or well composed, but they reveal the virtues of human beings, the relationships that are formed, and the set of chaotic and disorderly elements that pile up in clinical data, including those that are projected by own doctor.

The family doctor has a photo album, a computerized file, or simply a file where old photographs — old medical records — are saved. When we review our album of photographs some of them are recent and others older. It is as if time were crouched behind them to flood us with memories involving those images: odours, flavors, scents and feelings, problems, doubts, uncertainty, anger, contacts, joys, sorrows, work overload, misunderstandings. These leap on us while we are defenceless in front of all the lights and shadows that arise from the restored images; some of the patients are unknown, other are very close in our memories. This is a journey like any other; it has its surprises and its price, the difference being that on this trip we know that we have already been other than we currently are.

The practice of looking at old medical records — old photographs — is not trivial for the family doctor. In some cases it is a pleasure, it may be an act of nostalgia or of punishment — want to catch what we lost, what has been carried away by time. After reflecting on the past, sometime will be needed to recover from the gale that emerged from the stunning images of what we were or what the others were.

# References

Anderson R, Bury M (Editors). Living with Chronic Illness. The Experience of Patients and Their Families. London: Unwin Hyman; 1988.

August Sander/Michael Somoroff. Absence of Subject. Sirius Arts Centre, Cork, Ireland. April 18-June 1, 2014. http://absenceofsubject.com/michaelsomoroff/?ac=current.

Chéjov A. El Pabellón número 6.Madrid: Alianza Editorial; 1998.

Loxterkamp D. Saving Fred: what family practice means to medicine. *BMJ* 2000;321:1567-1568.

Margarit R. El río del tiempo. 12/02/2005.

Spiegel D. Living Beyond Limits. New Hope and Help for Facing Life-threatening Illness. London: Vermilion; 1993.

The New Yorker. The Emotion and Artifice of Medical Actors. JANUARY 2, 2016. http://www.newyorker.com/culture/photo-booth/the-emotion-and-artifice-of-medical-actors?mbid=nl_160104_Daily&CNDID=36284699&spMailingID=8397925&spUserID=OTg1NjczODA4NTMS1&spJobID=840351876&spReportId=ODQwMzUxODc2S0.

Tolstoy L. La muerte de Ivan Ilitch, Barcelona: Editorial Juventud, S.A.; 1984.

*Chapter 18*

# The Family Doctor as an Historian

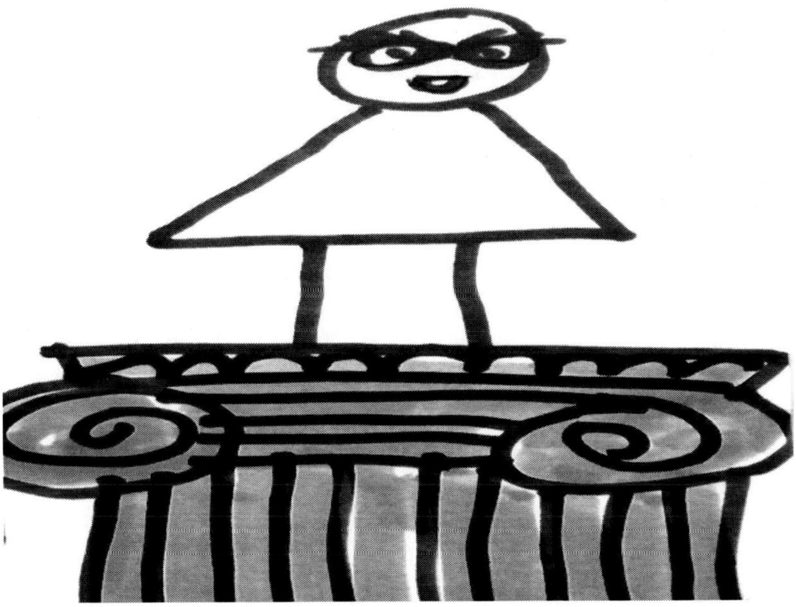

Why can be useful to family doctors in knowing the methods of the historian or the interpreter? Human life is a path through time, the historical route of a society with complex parts. The family doctor bases his work on an understanding of patients and their traces or data that allow us to reconstruct a history and predict a future. To create a proper history it is important to not only uncover the patient experience but also to expose the set of concepts or meanings that guide that experience.

The historian works with material remains or documents, with tracks or traces, real or imaginary, left by human beings and societies through time. These may lie in the landscape or in the basement, or in files located by the historian. In other words, to find them, interrogate them, and relate them to each other, the historian has first to look for those tracks. To know and use the methods of good historians may then be important for family doctors.

Historical research is conducted using "sources" through which "data" is derived to try to reconstruct the past. However, the sources and data do not contain a unique possibility of reading and interpretation but are encoded depending on who and how they are read, that is, there are no data are independent of a theoretical framework. In other words, the past that the historian interprets is not a fixed past but is one that moves according to the time from which the historian observes and the social perspective that he adopts — this can be thought of as similar to a landscape that moves according to the climber ascending to the summit. Therefore, even if we are not aware of it, we study and interpret the past from the concerns of the present and, at the same time, the present informs our interpretation of the past.

In addition, the present is not univocal, but it criss-crossed by several tensions that result from the clash of multiple interests. What perspective should the historian choose? Can an historian be objective? The mission of the historian is to collect the preserved stories or testimonials, and examine and interpret them to determine their meaning and validity. The notion of objectivity is an unattainable illusion worshipped by positivist historians. Pure objectivity is a fiction. The historian is part of the history he studies and cannot (though he may wish to) put aside his subjectivity when he tries to meet his object of study. Subjectivity is inherent in the process of knowledge and, therefore, is not something bad that emerges from it. It becomes bad only when the historian allows his interests and biases distort the knowledge that he aspires to build.

The historian interprets, evaluates and judges from the beginning of his work until he its completion. He uses value judgements when he has to decide which of the available sources he is going to use. He judges when he has to choose between one or another fact, between one and another process to emphasize the point more or less clearly. When he has to explain a course of events using little evidence, he chooses to interpret the findings in a meaningful context that, according to his reason, offers a compelling sense of the past. The historian must be equipped with a theoretical and conceptual framework that facilitates the organization and analysis of data and gives meaning to the past. The theoretical concepts are the instruments par excellence that allow the historian to define the facts and select, within the virtual infinity of the past data, those that are most important and relevant.

History cannot be understood if the historian fails to establish any contact with the minds of those on which he works. We can only achieve capture and understanding of the past through the lens of the present. History is a continuum between the historian and the facts, and through endless dialogue between the present and the past. From a methodological perspective, the historian must be highly flexible and reflective in the treatment of the data.

If the discipline of clinical medicine can be related to the discipline of history, doctors must learn the working methods of the historian. The needs of the current empirical clinic cannot be achieved by the didactic methods of the past. With constant changes in the nature of contemporary clinical problems, the information necessary for the clinical features, and the responsibilities of the family doctor should be accompanied by changes in educational methods. The educational goal is to train family doctors in how to discover the facts located within the sick or healthy patient and to include them in the diagnostic and therapeutic process via an egalitarian collaboration with the information about disease, physiopathology and technology. Perhaps some training in the tasks and methods of the historian may be helpful to the family doctor.

# References

Churchill Jr. CJ. Ethnography as Translation. *Qualitative Sociology*. 2005; 28(1): 3–24.
Helman CG. *Culture, Health and Illness*. Oxford: Butterworth Heinemann Ltd; 1994.
Turabian JL. El médico de familia como historiador e intérprete. JANO 2005; LXVIII(1.553):10.

*Chapter 19*

# The Family Doctor as a Person Eating Spaghetti or Cherries

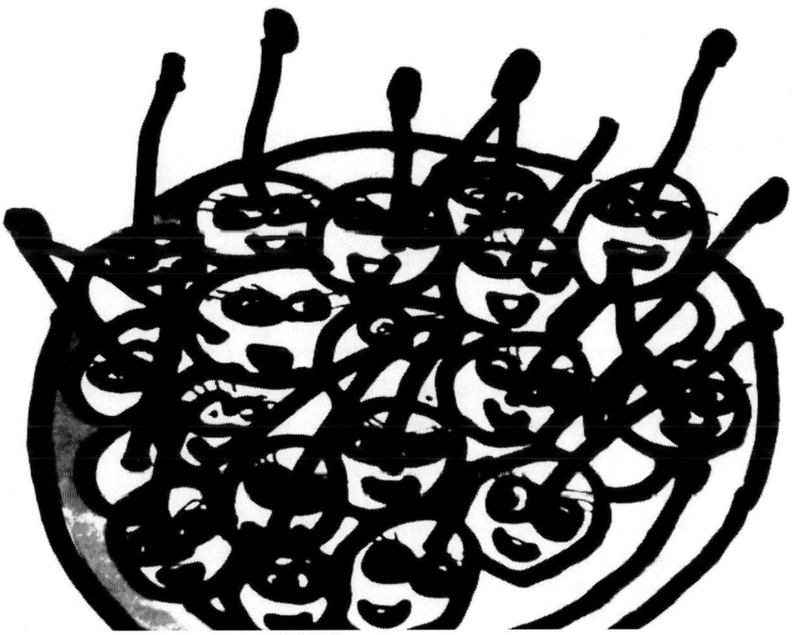

The family doctor may know the correct way to eat spaghetti, the proper way — trying not to splash tomato on his face and his shirt and trying to get the right amount of food into his mouth — but he may not get it right. Although family physicians may use a fork and spoon, not even being Italian, he fails.

When the family doctor sees a patient who consults for a problem, he cannot focus only on that problem since other problems (that are glued to each other). This is akin to picking cherries from a basket: they are hooked to each other and tangled together by the ends, making it impossible to pull out one without taking many more.

Classical epidemiological chains essentially depend on factors that influence the likelihood of contact between the infectious agent and the susceptible person (the host). For example, a person has tuberculosis because his weak body was penetrated by Mycobacterium tuberculosis. Thus, the classic epidemiological triad is built on three illars: agent (more or less virulent), human host (more or less resistant), and environment (more or less favourable). However, this triad has limitations because sometimes the agent or cause is intrinsic to the host or environment and, above all, because there are factors in the chain that are behind the agent: these are the "causes of the agent."

So, to the family doctor, the lack of health can be seen as the apex of a pyramid: at its apex is the pathology (e.g., ischemic heart disease). But physiological risk factors (hypercholesterolemia) lie below, and behavioral risk factors (diet) are even lower. The latter are due to factors that are even lower in the pyramid (values and meanings), and these are due to those further down (social norms and customs), which, in turn, these are due to those below (trade practices, regulations, cultural values, free markets, the unrealistic dependence on the health system). Doctors have been attentive to the apex of the pyramid: the diagnosis and treatment of disease. Doctors see the physiological risks that result in the chemical and physiological parameters of disease but they neglect the behavioral factors and background circumstances.

Socio-economic status is a powerful determinant of health. Although wages, education and profession, in all probability, do not directly affect health, they have indirect effects through other variables. These include smoking, alcohol consumption, substance abuse, trauma, diet, stress, exposure to infectious or toxic agents and so on — all factors that tend to be more frequently associated with socially disadvantaged groups. These social-economic factors may prove to be immeasurably more important than "the causes" of ill health. The social environment is the main or primary determinant of health and disease in any community. Life is a complex system, it is nonlinear, without conditions of normality, and is independence of variables.

The cause of ill health is not a one-way action from the outer to the inner or from the internal to the external, but is an interaction thereof that necessarily involves an effect, and a cause and an effect that are constantly changing places, interacting, and forming connections.

The family doctor knows this "epidemiology of cherries in a basket and eating spaghetti effect" and so knows that when he gets to a certain level of the pyramid of causes it is somewhat arbitrary or based on the feasibility of the decision and, if he pulls, a little bit of "spaghetti" appears with more causes that are increasingly important, and the clothes of the doctor become splashed with tomato.

## References

J. L. Turabián, S. Moreno-Ruiz y R. Cucho-Jove. "Doctor, tengo Chikungunya." Sistematización conceptual de las implicaciones epidemiológicas específicas desde la medicina de familia. *Semergen.* 2015. http://www.elsevier.es/es-revista--40-linkresolver-doctor-tengo-chikungunya-sistematizacion-conceptual-S11383593(15)003160.

Miguel García F. Factores de riesgo: una nada inocente ambigüedad en el corazón de la medicina actual. *Aten Primaria* 1998; 22(9):585-595.

Milne V, Laupacis A, Tierney M. Are family doctors cherry picking patients? *Healthy Debate.* October 23, 2014. http://healthydebate.ca/2014/10/topic/family-doctors-cherry-picking-patients.

Sagatovsky, V.N. y Antipov, I.G. Acerca de la correlación entre los conceptos "causa," "condición." "etiología" y "pathogenesis." *Vestu Akad Med Nauk* 1966. 21:34-40.

Selva Sutter E. Más allá de Sagatovski y Antipov: La causalidad estructural puntualizada. Universidad Centroamericana José Simeón Cañas. Departamento de Salud Pública. Maestría en Salud Pública. San Salvador, febrero de 1999. http://www.uca.edu.sv/facultad/chn/sagindice.html.

Tarlov AR. The rising supply of physicians and the pursuit of better health. *Journal of Medical Education*, 1988; 63: 94-107.

*Chapter 20*

# The Family Doctor as a Translator

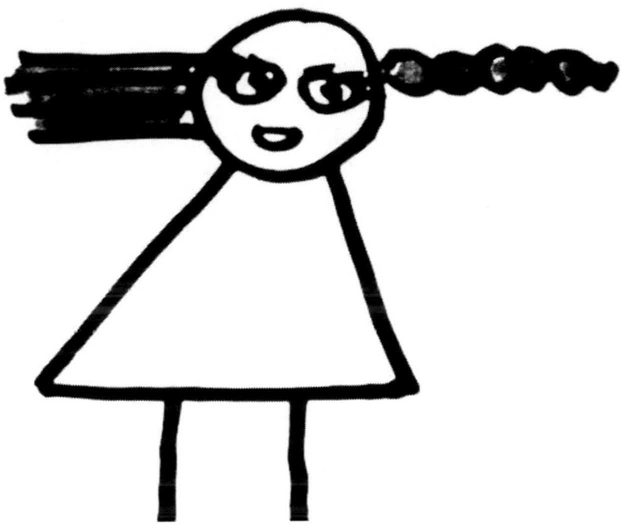

The family doctor is like a translator. He has to translate from one language to another: from the language of the patient to the language of science. This requires that the translator fully understands "the meaning and matter" that he translates. It is necessary that he has a perfect knowledge of the language of the author that he translates and, equally, of the language into which he is translating — in the translation it is not necessary to convert the text word by word. Those who make this mistake frequently distort the sense of the author and do not express the grace and perfection of either of the languages.

Family medicine is a form of translation in order to clarify what occurs between the data acquisition and the development of diagnosis and treatment of these data. The patient speaks in a strange language and we have to translate it and check our translation ("if I understand correctly, the pain started three days ago ... and then ran to ... and a fever appeared ...?").

The mind of the family doctor should be seen as a transitional space which, in the act of translating field data into an analytical diagnosis (1) poses a unique challenge to provide an exact vision of the patient's situations, while (2) simultaneously, providing pathways for the patient, his context and his health problem, that the qualitative and quantitative research cannot give separately.

On the streets of Bialystok you can hear Yiddish, Polish, Hebrew, Belarusian, German, and Russian — Esperanto was invented by a student in that city. Perhaps the family doctor should do a rotation in the different "departments" of Bialystok!

## References

Bittner A, Bittner J, Jonietz A, Dybowski C, Harendza S. Translating medical documents improves students' communication skills in simulated physician-patient encounters. BMC Medical Education. 2016; 16:72. http://bmcmededuc.biomedcentral.com/articles/10.1186/s12909-016-0594-4.

Burgess A. La naranja mecánica. Barcelona: Minoauro; 1988.

Churchill Jr. CJ. Ethnography as Translation. *Qualitative Sociology.* 2005¸ 28(1): 3 – 24.

Neighbourg R. The inner consultation. Lancaster: MTP press; 1991.

Salomé J, Galland S. Si me escuchara, me entendería. Santander: Sal Terrae;1996.

Turabián Fernández JL, Pérez Franco B. Notes on "resolutivity" and "cure" in family medicine. Aten Primaria. 2003; 32:296-9. http://www.elsevier.es/es-revista-atencion-primaria-27-articulo-apuntes-resolutividad-cura-medicina-familia-13051598.

Turabian JL. Cuadernos de Medicina de Familia y Comunitaria. Diaz de SAntos SA. Madrid 1995:198-226.

*Chapter 21*

# The Family Doctor as an Ethnographer

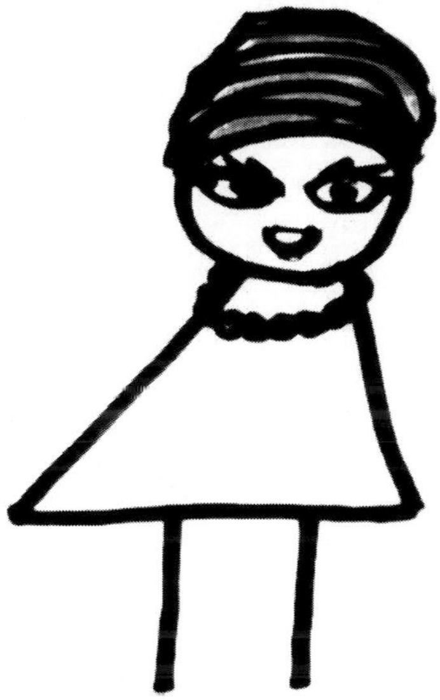

A look at the activities in the daily life of the family doctor shows great similarities between qualitative research and its practice. The experience of being a family doctor is similar to that of being an ethnographer who carries out a qualitative study. The family doctor works in the same surgery for a long time, developing relationships with his patients and their contexts, and realizing their visions and knowledge. In this way the doctor is able to better interpret the signs and symptoms of the diseases that these people present. In the surgery, the family doctor as an ethnographer conducts an interview with a patient and, for this, he needs to establish empathy and to try to understand and interpret the perspective, experience, feelings and values of the patient. As an ethnographer, the family doctor has to interact with a great variety of people, many of who have different ways of understanding reality and vastly different stories and life experiences. Both family doctor and ethnographer negotiate their relationships with these different people in order to minimize the barriers to comprehension. But, unlike the ethnographer, the family doctor is orientated to practice and must therefore treat every patient.

Beyond being an experimenter, the family doctor should be naturalist. To do so, he must look through the eyes of a researcher to see the nature of the pain that is presented to him. We rarely remember that many more than fifty per cent of modern medicine is due to the simple and pure observation of the pathological and its correct interpretation. There are doctors who, after many years of practice, have not found a single new detail to add to those described in the pathology books. There are surgeons with copious numbers of operations in all classes who, in spite of the experiment that is every surgery, have not seen anything new. Those that have not thought of modifying an instrument or inventing new other one, are absent to a basic duty, are improper usufructuaries of the science. They may make excuses such as, "we have not contributed to the truth because we were unable to investigate." Yet the truth is not only to be found in the experiment but also in the simple and fecund observation.

The clinic is an enigmatic and particular combination of concept and experience. We know from own experience that there are some problems that the patient communicates quickly, but there are others that remain hidden. At least a third of patients in primary care have psychosocial problems that they perceive as influencing their health situation/disease. The family doctor, however, is aware of only a fraction of these psychosocial problems of their patients, depending on the type of problem, prior knowledge of the patient and the patient's socio-demographic characteristics. The variations in the patients' desire to communicate these problems, and the skills with which they are able to do so, depend on the need for trust in the doctor-patient relationship before they feel able to reveal intimate problems. The tendency of the doctors and primary care professionals to limit their expectations may also be a reason for the low detection of psychosocial problems in primary care.

Thinking is a way of exploring our maps of accumulated experiences; it is like exploring the street map of a city. Some routes are familiar, others show us shortcuts, and sometimes we can see the start but not the right route. Using our "stock" of solutions and applying them according to the experience is the role of the doctor.

## References


Crane JG, Angrosino MV. Field projects in antropology. Illinois: Waveland Pres Inc; 1992.

Dubos R. Celebraciones de la vida. Mexico: Fondo de Cultura Económica; 1985.

Gannik DE. Situational disease. *Fam Pract* 1995;12:202-206.

Goenka S. A day in the field that changed my methodology. *BMJ* 2002;324:493. http://www.bmj.com/content/324/7335/493.1.full.

http://www.amazon.es/Actividades-comunitarias-medicina-atenci%C3%B3n-primaria/dp/8479784741.

Marañón G. La medicina y nuestro tiempo. Madrid: Espasa Calpe; 1980.

Rogers CR. A way of being. New York: Houghton Mifflin Company; 1995.

Turabian JL, Pérez Franco B. Actividades Comunitarias en Medicina de Familia y Atención Primaria. Madrid: Díaz de Santos; 2001.

William James. The varieties of religious experience, 1958.

*Chapter 22*

# The Family Doctor as a Cat

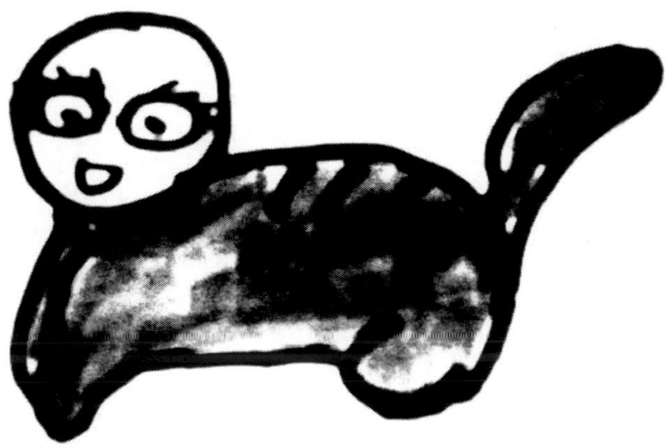

Cats have seven lives. There is no doubt that the exceptional strength of the cat, its ability to emerge unscathed from complicated situations or to jump considerable heights without suffering the least damage when other animals may have died, suggests that these animals have more than one life. A lucky person has seven lives, like cats. Family physicians are lucky because they have nine lives!

Like cats, family physicians fall on their feet. The constitution of the cat's spine is such that it allows them to make a twisting motion and to rotate themselves in the air and land on their feet. The bio-psychosocial perspective of family doctors allows them to "turn on themselves."

Like cats, family physicians need to think and act before they have all the necessary information. To deal with ill-defined health problems and diseases in their early stages of evolution, the family doctor needs a bio-psychosocial vision, unlike the hospital physician who can take a strictly biomedical view of illness.

In addition, the family doctor, as the cat, has top rate senses of smell and hearing, in many respects greater than those of other specialists. The "ears" of the family doctor "can rotate 180 degrees," like those of the cat, so that they can scan the area and assess with high accuracy, the problems, actors, and contexts around them.

In addition, family physicians and cats have an excellent sense of direction. Thus, in caring for the patient the family doctor can simultaneously view the information derived from the context in which the patient has symptoms, and their prior knowledge of the patient (continuity of care). As a result, the doctor decides the severity of the problem and makes a diagnosis.

Consequently, perhaps family doctors have to learn to purr.

# References

Balint JA. Brief Encounters: Speaking with Patients. *Ann Intern Med.* 1999; 131: 231-234. http://www.annals.org/cgi/reprint/131/3/231.pdf.

Engel GJ. The need for a new medical model: a challenge for biomedicine. *Science.* 1977; 196(4286): 129-136. http://www.sciencemag.org/cgi/content/abstract/196/4286/129.

Engel GL. The clinical application of the biopsychosocial model. *Am J Psychiatry* 1980; 137:535-544.

http://ajp.psychiatryonline.org/cgi/content/abstract/137/5/535?ijkey=3a1702d8ae52851716e2636cd0560b178a5fb272&keytype2=tf_ipsecsha.

Sanders k. Nine lives. The emocional experience in general practice. Worcester: Clunie Press for The Rolond Harris Trust Library. Monograph series Nº 5; 1991.

*Chapter 23*

# The Family Doctor as a Civil Engineer

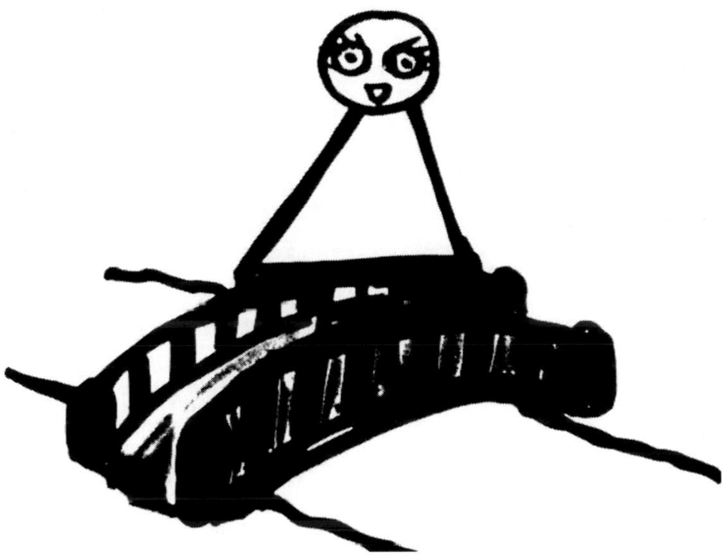

When on vacation, some doctors are asked their profession by their neighbors. To avoid being asked about symptoms, medication and so on, some say that they are "engineers." These doctors say it as a joke, but the truth is they are correct; most family physicians are "civil engineers."

The task of the family doctor is to build bridges (civil engineer!) between himself (with his knowledge and contexts) and the patients (with their beliefs, concerns, experiences and contexts), to find a point where they can "pass" or "cross the bridge." These bridges result in agreements for the maintenance of the relationship and for achieving collaborations that enable the patients to move forward.

Medicine is not only for the sick person; it can help you stay on a path. Here the crucial task of the family doctor is to build a path for health. This not only involves the resources of modern medicine but also the effect of doctor himself and the whole personality and context of the patient.

The diagnosis in family medicine "comes to the end." The first is the treatment ("build bridges"), and after this we can make the diagnosis. The purpose of the family doctor is to provide the conditions (being a civil engineer) in which the patient is able to experience and accept the diagnosis of the problem areas.

One of the main tasks of the doctor is to enable the patients to mobilize their full potential, their own strengths, and the potential of both their bodies and minds against the disease. For precisely this reason, the family doctor builds bridges and roads that are suitable for the patient.

The family doctor should pay attention to the psychology of the patient, regardless of the diagnosis of the disease, if he wants the patient to recover. The psychology of the seriously ill may place barriers between him and his medical skills, and building bridges across these hiatuses is required. There is a feeling of hopelessness in cases of serious disease. Patients fears they will never regain their normal functions and this produces a barrier separating the sick from a world of wide expectations and choices.

Today, medicine suffers from an abundance of resources and a poverty of goals. Medicine is increasingly separated from the direction of human life; it has become a monolithic discipline that talks in terms of of health and autonomy but continues to define everything in terms of biomedical pathology. Family physicians must build bridges and roads if we are to achieve a human-sized healthcare.

## References

http://www.amazon.co.uk/Cuadernos-medicina-familia-y-comunitaria/dp/8479781920.

Jensen W. Gradiva. Una fantasía pompeyana. Barcelona: Ediciones La Tempestad; 2005.

Turabian JL. Cuadernos de Medicina de Familia y Comunitaria. Una introducción a los principios de Medicina de Familia. Madrid: Díaz de Santos. 1995.

Turabian JL. El médico de familia es un "ingeniero de caminos." *JANO*. 2003; LXIV (1.465): 544. http://www.jano.es/ficheros/sumarios/1/64/1465/10/1v64n1465a13044201pdf001.pdf.

Chapter 24

# The Family Doctor as a Film Director

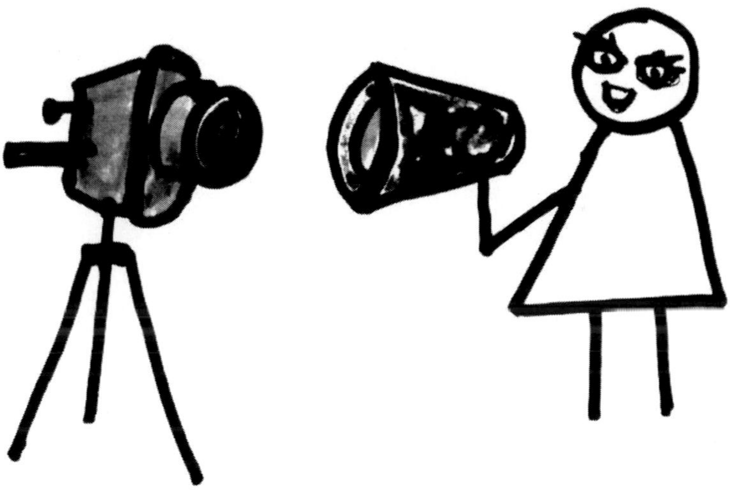

The filmmaker or film director is the person who directs the making of a film, gives instructions to the actors, who makes decisions about the location of the camera monitors, the scenery, the costumes, and all other functions necessary to bring the film to fruition. A film is a cinematic masterpiece that, in an audio-visual manner, tells a story or a fact. The film is constituted by a sequence of images. From the technical point of view, a movie is a string of photographic images taken with a camera and reproduced using a projector.

You can compare the process in family medicine to a film in which the episode of illness is like a scene from a movie, and the family physician knows that these sequences are simply parts of a whole. Successful clinical decisions should be driven by a set of tests, values, or preferences and circumstances.

In the context of the consultation in family medicine, where unpredictable changes occur, the ability of the family doctor to act both with confidence and with full knowledge of the uncertainty is based on being able to look ahead and consider uncertainties, as in the scenes and the script of a film. In addition, some "staging" or organization of the performance space with the patient occurs during the clinical interview, as it does in a movie.

The "scenarios/scripts" are stories about the way the patient might experience tomorrow, stories that can help us realize and adapt to the changing aspects of our current context. The scenarios/scripts are a way to articulate the different paths that might exist for us in the future, and to find an appropriate path through each possible move. Scenario planning is about taking decisions and making choices today with an understanding of how things might change in the future.

Scenarios recall a set of stories or narratives, both written and spoken, as in a movie. Scenarios can help people plan future decisions and, often, tough choices that otherwise might be lost or hidden.

There is also a "movie" of interpersonal continuity in the family doctor's office. As in a film, different scenes appear and over time there may be changes of light and scenarios. Thus, over time, some of our patients disappear and not only because they die. There are also those who, over a long or short period have apparently been satisfied patients, there are those who vanish into a remote limbo, new patients arrive, new challenges appear, and so on. The film will continue.

## References

Anja Kapmeyer, Christoph Meyer, Michael M Kochen, and Wolfgang Himme. Doctors' strategies in prescribing drugs: the case of mood-modifying Medicines. l. *Fam. Pract.* 2006 23: 73-79. http://fampra.oxfordjournals.org/cgi/content/abstract/23/1/73?etoc.

Eisenstein SM. El sentido del cine. Buenos Aires, Argentina: Siglo XXI Argentina Editores S.A.; 1974.

Landstrom B; Rudebeck CE; Mattsson B. Working behaviour of competent general practitioners: Personal styles and deliberate strategies. *Scand J Prim Health Care* 2006 Jun;24(2):122-8. http://www.ncbi.nlm.nih.gov/pubmed/16690562.

Olesen F, Dickinson J, Hjortdahl P. General practice—time for a new definition. *BMJ* 2000; 320:326-327. http://www.bmj.com/content/320/7231/354.full.

Schwartz P. The art of the long view. New York: Doubleday; 1991.

Turabián Fernández JL, Pérez Franco B. Una forma de hacer operativo el pragmatismo clínico: sistematización del modo de acción de los médicos competentes. *Med Clin* (Barc) 2005;124:476. http://www.elsevier.es/es-revista-medicina-clinica-2-articulo-una-forma-hacer-operativo-el-13073233.

Turabián JL, Pérez Franco B. Critically examining the symptoms and diagnoses that are taken for granted in family medicine. creating an own school. *Semergen.* 2012;38(2):67-71. http://www.elsevier.es/es-revista-semergen-medicina-general-familia-40-articulo-examinando-criticamente-los-sintomas-diagnosticos-que-se-90108498.

Turner J, Pugh J, Budiani D. "It's Always Continuing": First-Year Medical Students' Perspectives on Chronic Illness and the Care of Chronically Ill Patients. *Acad Med.* 2005; 80(2):183-8. http://www.ncbi.nlm.nih.gov/pubmed/15671326.

*Chapter 25*

# The Family Doctor as a Tourist That Opens a Folded Map

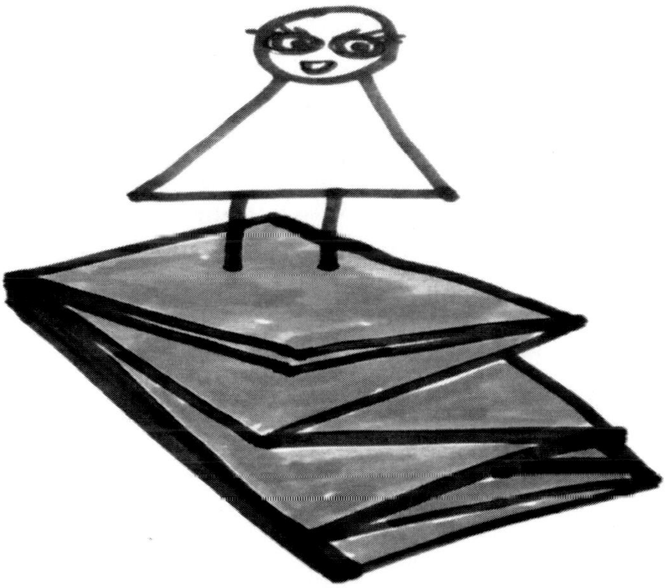

The diagnosis in family medicine involves deploying a map that allows a panoramic vision.

A diagnosis in the model of family medicine can be seen as a map. The map uses certain standard schemes as the contours, the symbols of roads, rivers, and bridges. These symbols are similar on all maps but each map is built to a scale. The map is useful but it is necessary to know its scale. Similarly, for the family doctor, a diagnosis of a fractured femur is certainly a fractured femur, but its significance in scale depends on the landscape or context. In the model that focuses only on the disease, the broken femur is a broken femur and nothing else.

In family medicine there is a tendency to think in terms of individual patients in their particular environments rather than abstractions and generalizations. Family physicians have difficulty separating the illness from the person who has it. The ideal is to integrate the particular and the general, to see the universal in the particular (the map and the territory).

To make an accurate diagnosis the family doctor must "deploy" a multisystem model, or an "open map" that integrates the various levels of the patient's condition to allow for the proper selection of the road down which the treatment should go. However this integration is difficult. The analysis, coordination, integration and implementation of this knowledge within a bio-psychosocial intervention is difficult. But this is what characterizes the family doctor, and you have to learn to do it.

For example, the impact of a disease such as type 2 diabetes mellitus occurs at very different levels. A doctor who does not display the map retains a biomedical vision and focuses on the lowest possible levels of systemic organization (molecules, cells, tissues, organs and organ systems), whereas by opening the map a family doctor opens a whole range of possible approaches, preferably focusing on the highest possible levels of systemic organization (family, community, culture, society).

When compared with the biological approach, which has, for example, to interpret MRI images (which requires a high level of skill), it is more difficult and requires more experience for a family doctor to "display the map" as the real difficulty is emotional. This difficulty speaks of fear of the emotional experience and transforms the problem into a mechanical or commercial transaction where the patient is a machine that can be studied. The understanding of human problems only comes from emotional experience, and this also requires the map to be displayed.

Family doctors gets to know their patients over time (their biographies, their expectations, their desires, their lives) and so, when the patient returns to the office the initial simple problem is taken as a starting point. However, when the map is opened a lot of connections and relationships are displayed that are helpful for the full understanding of the problem, its diagnosis, and therapeutic intervention.

## References

Gannik DE. Situational disease. Fam Pract 1995; 12:202-206. http://fampra.oxfordjournals.org/content/12/2/202.abstract.

Turabian JL, Pérez Franco B. Actividades Comunitarias en Medicina de Familia y Atención Primaria. Madrid: Díaz de Santos; 2001. http://www.amazon.es/Actividades-comunitarias-medicina-atenci%C3%B3n-primaria/dp/8479784741.

Turabián JL, Pérez Franco B. The diagnostic concept in family medicine: A view of the landscape. The diagnosis in family medicine. Aten Primaria. 2010. http://www.elsevier.es/revistas/ctl_servlet?_f=7064&articuloid=13146911&revistaid=27&ip=85.48.234.32&redir_user_contactid=QzJKUjRBMDA5ODNP.

Van Swaaij L, Klare J. The Atlas of Experience. London: Bloonsbury Publishing Plc.; 2000.

Vicenzi A. (Editor)La Galería de los Mapas en el Vaticano. Modena, Italy: Franco Cosimo Panini Editore SPA.; 2012.

*Chapter 26*

# The Family Doctor as an Architect

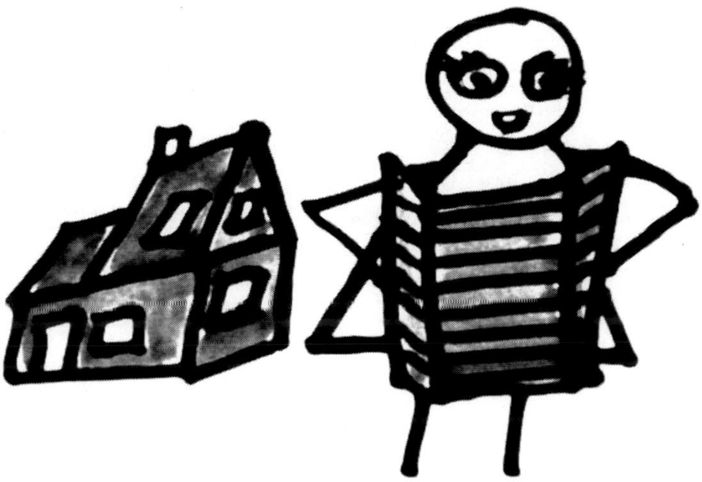

Conception and birth, growth and maturity, aging and death — these are important moments in the human life story. They are also stages in the existence of a building. We can apply the metaphor of a life cycle to buildings, extending it to the phases of birth, maturity, and death to include the rituals that often accompany these stages. Many of us can connect a personal life experience, such as graduation, to "the life rituals of constructed forms," such as a ground-breaking cornerstone ceremony, and milestone anniversaries. Like the architect, the family doctor attempts to endow patients or buildings with a healthy personality. Both the family doctor and the architect have debates over the naming of diseases or buildings, and the attempts to document the erection and aging of buildings. The family doctor and the architect attempt to prolong building's life and vitality, and both are concerned with "sick" and endangered buildings. Also, both experience the difficulty that people have in saying goodbye to old buildings or to patients who feel like friends.

Building a private building, such as a home, affects the lives of many others: the neighbor whose garden in its shadow, the children who grow up in it, the people maintain it as it ages, and all those who bear the impact of the resources consumed and the pollution emitted. And the building lasts for a long time, so its potential impacts branch through the generations.

Similarly, interventions by general practitioners, whose work is directed toward an individual, have powerful effects on others: family, work, relationships, and community context.

As architects, family physicians need to be aware that there are others whose needs will be affected by any intervention and that only the family doctor can defend this. It is the balance between of all these considerations that serves all these groups. The architect cannot ignore the enormous value of the community, the local knowledge and local ties. He also has to develop and keep in mind an intimate understanding of the local climate, topography, history, social dynamics, and building traditions.

An architect should be able to advise a client about a place or building that may be attractive at first sight but could be unusually exposed to the fog and winter storms.

The architect should also take note of what materials and design details work best in a particular cultural environment or physical environment. These rules also apply to the family doctor, who needs to know the community. Good health allows us to connect with family and neighbors in the consolidation of relations. When disease is present this can lead to loneliness, resignation and despair.

Each building presents opportunities to promote or prevent healthy, positive relationships, and connections with the environment. It is the job of the architect to identify these opportunities and, as far as possible, to aim their work in the right direction. The difference between alienation and connection depends not only on social and economic forces, but also on countless "micro" incidents such as those that occur when two neighbors are chatting on the sidewalk, when a family talks at the table after dinner, when a child who falls asleep to the sound of its parents' voices outside porch. The architecture works on this scale of experience. In family medicine tasks carried out at a small calibre level can subtly tilt the world towards dignity, compassion, and health.

## References

Harris N. Building Lives: Constructing Rites and Passages. New Haven and London: Yale University Press; 1999.

Loxterkamp D, Snider B. What doctors have in common with architects—part 1: A manual art. *BMJ* 2015;350:h1810. http://www.bmj.com/content/350/bmj.h1810?etoc=.

Loxterkamp D, Snider B. What doctors have in common with architects—part 2: The common good. *BMJ* 2015;350:h1823. http://www.bmj.com/content/350/bmj.h1823?etoc=.

*Chapter 27*

# The Family Doctor as a Catalyst

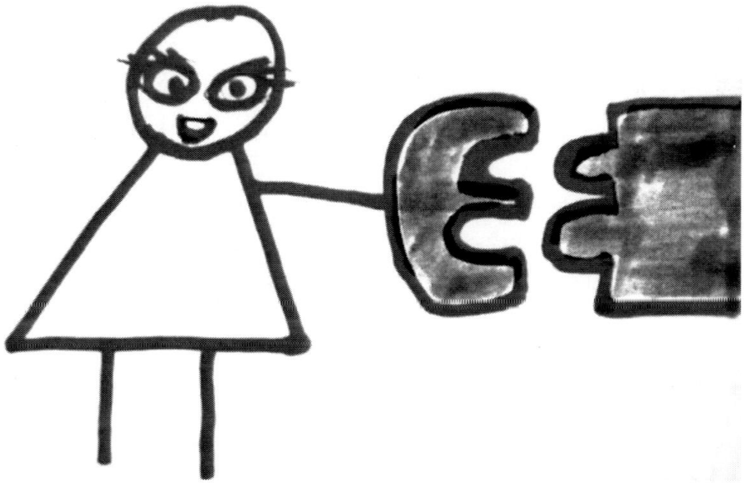

The family doctor is like a "catalyst" in chemistry.

Catalysts are chemicals that are not directly involved in the chemical reaction but they make it faster and, in some cases, enhance the final quality.

The family physician is a catalyst: a small amount, when present in the chemical reaction, can produce great results. So the family doctor continuously performs interventions called "small interventions," such as minimal interventions for smoking cessation, psychotherapy, and so on, which are actually "major" in terms of their effects. At first glance the family physician is a small enzyme that appears insignificant but which depends on the pace and speed of a chemical reaction. There are thousands of specific enzymes to thousands of chemical reactions. Our task is a minimal, humble task, but is very important: to discover what stands between people's health and their ability to attain it, and to achieved this using minimal effort – thus encouraging the individual to be in a better position to move forward.

The work of the family doctor resembles a powerful reagent. Their presence is never overbearing, it is always prudent and adapted to the requirements of each situation, and is evidenced in the speed and quality of the results.

# References

Balint E, Norell JS (Ed). Six minutes for the patient: interactions in general practice consultations. London: Tavistock publications; 1973.

http://www.amazon.es/Actividades-comunitarias-medicina-atenci%C3%B3n-primaria/dp/8479784741.

Turabian JL, Pérez Franco B. Actividades Comunitarias en Medicina de Familia y Atención Primaria. Madrid: Díaz de Santos; 2001.

Turabián JL, Pérez-Franco B. Which is the goal of health education and "community" activities in primary care? *Aten Primaria* 1998; 22(10):662-666. http://www.elsevier.es/es-revista-atencion-primaria-27-articulo-cual-es-el-sentido-educacion-14992.

*Chapter 28*

# The Family Doctor as an Impressionist Painter

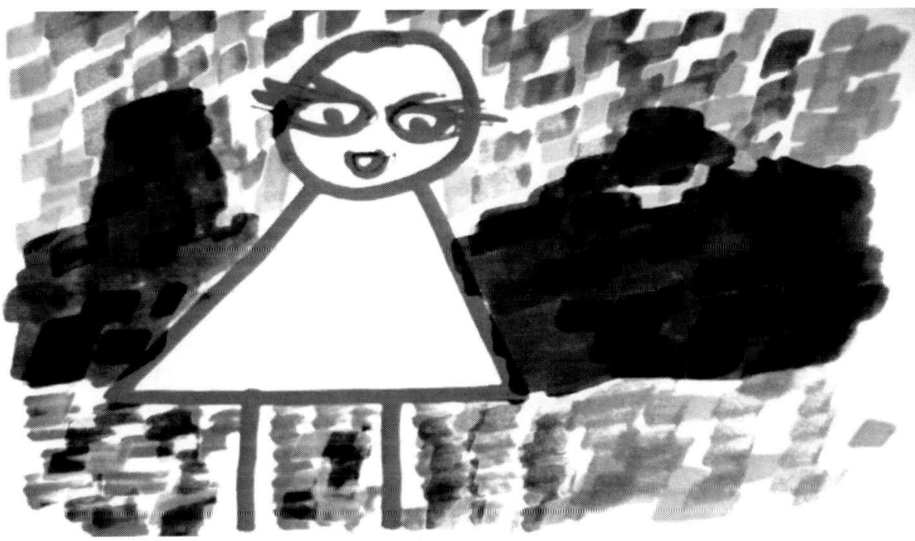

The family physician develops a way to look like an impressionist painter. These painters were not concerned with the composition of objects but with the impact the environment had on them. According to impressionism there are as many different landscapes of the same scene as the day has moments. That is exactly the opposite of what is meant by "realism" which caters only to the object and its invariance, without the impact the environment has on the object.

The scientist chooses to know things in themselves, regardless of the circumstances. The scientific work style is an abstraction of context (an abstraction of particular case). In each "objective" thing the scientists consider only the contextual considerations that most interest them. Here the family doctor is the opposite of "scientific": attempting to know things in the circumstances, contextualizing.

The painter must, in one way or another, solve the hierarchical relationship between things and space: he does this by giving the same interest to the two factors, giving prominence to either one or the other. The fact that things depend on the environment is the essential characteristic of impressionism. When, conversely, the environment is sacrificed to the representation of particular objects, we see an anti-impressionist art, which we may call classical art. A Monet and a Greek vessel with painted figures indicate the two extremes: the first appear to be immersed in the environment; individuality and contours do not already exist. In the second, the figures on a Greek vessel, the landscape or the environment appears to be totally sacrificed.

## References

D'Ors E. Pablo Picasso en tres revisiones. Barcelona: ABC, S.L.; 2003.

Sopena JM, Romero E. Neural netwroks and lineal methods in medical diagnosis: relevance of irrelevant variables. Med Clin (Barc) 122(9):336-338, 2004. http://www.elsevier.es/en-revista-medicina-clinica-2-articulo-redes-neuronales-metodos-estadisticos-clasicos-13059028.

Gannik DE. Situational disease. Fam Pract 12(2):202-206, 1995. http://fampra.oxfordjournals.org/content/12/2/202.abstract.

*Chapter 29*

# The Family Doctor as a Wizard

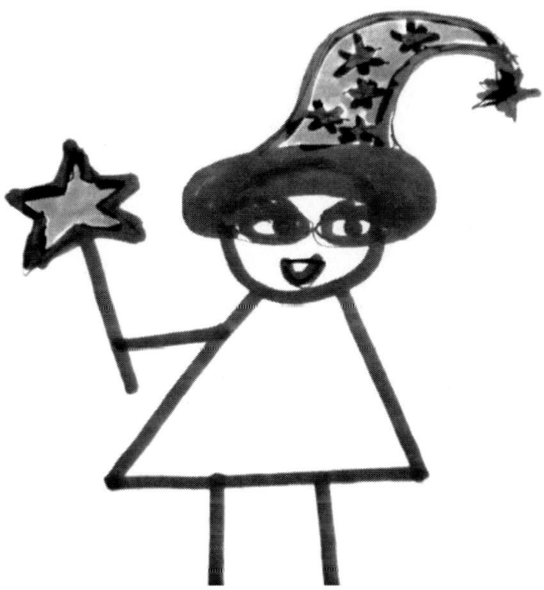

The family doctor sees a patient in ten minutes, during which time a diagnosis is made and treatment is performed. For a novice observer, such as a medical student or a resident, this is incomprehensible, it's magic! It's like pulling a rabbit out of the hat. But we need to know the trick if we are to be able to repeat it. How does the family doctor make these diagnoses appear or disappear and how does he guess the thoughts of the patient? Maybe he studies the stars and reads crystal balls?

The meaning of "art" or "clinical expertise" is associated with the ability or capacity to manage the uncertainty of the problem. Trying to negate the "old" concept of "clinical eye of the wise physician" (subjectively) to emphasize clinical epidemiology (objectively) as a unique approach is a mistake in the development of the family doctor.

The clinical emerges, that is, it is perceived by the clinician within a theoretical framework that clarifies the reality. From that moment, there are a number of clinical strategies to manage the uncertainty of decision-making: the internal consistency of the doctor, congruence with other stakeholders, the internal consistency of semiotics, and temporal consistency. Each of these strategies has a number of clinical techniques.

From the paradigm of positivist science (quantitative, objective) the clinician primarily uses clinical strategies to manage uncertainty, clinical epidemiology, and evidence based medicine. But many other techniques are frequently used. These techniques are the "tricks of the magician" and they are qualitative techniques such as contextualization, experience, continuity of care, common sense, strategic planning, use of resources and strengths, self-esteem, self-efficacy, emotion, intuition, ethics, the participation of patients and communities, the use of our senses, the test of time, compassion, ecological and networked relations, focusing on the process rather than the outcome, the clinical interview and empathy, efficiency and effectiveness, creativity, and so on.

The family doctor is a magician in the sense of being wise, that is, someone with the ability to see what others do not see, to feel what, for most people, passes unnoticed — the trick is to use these powerful subjective tools.

## References

De Bono E. *Textbook of wisdow*. London: Penguin Books; 1996.

Marín R, De la Torre S. (Coordinadores). Manual de la Creatividad. Aplicaciones educativas. Barcelona: Vicens Vives; 1991.

Shaw B. The Doctor's dilemma. Edinburgh: Penguin Books; 1958.

Turabián Fernández JL, Pérez Franco B. Una forma de hacer operativo el pragmatismo clínico: sistematización del modo de acción de los médicos competentes. Med Clin (Barc) 2005;124:476. http://www.elsevier.es/es-revista-medicina-clinica-2-articulo-una-forma-hacer-operativo-el-13073233.

Turabián JL, Pérez Franco B. A way to make clinical pragmatism operative: sistematization of the actuation of competent physicians. *Med Clin* (Bar) 2005;124(12):476. http://www.elsevier.es/es-revista-medicina-clinica-2-articulo-una-forma-hacer-operativo-el-13073233.

*Chapter 30*

# The Family Doctor as a Fisherman with a Hook

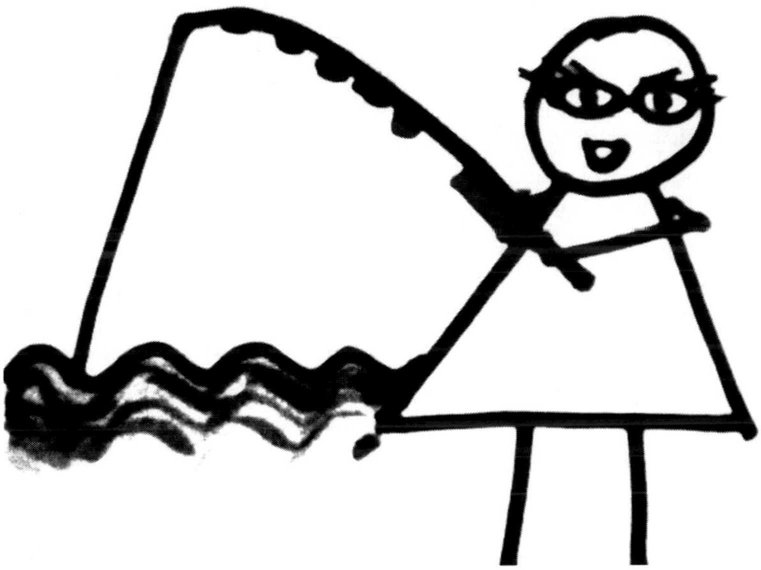

Confucius said that "the Master did not fish with a net, but with a hook."

There is a debate between small-scale traditional techniques — the hook — and techniques for large-scale fishing, or industrial overfishing, which will eventually worsen the health of the sea and bring negative consequences for the people who live from it. From the epidemiological point of view, the family doctor has at least five reasons to go fishing with a hook and to avoid the network of massive fishing, with the problematic consequences that the latter brings.

1. The method in family medicine is to identify pre-symptomatic disease or screening — the fishing network. This is undertaken through "case-findings" — fishing with a hook. The activities of screening a cohort, where the service is offered to a selected group within the population, it is replaced for of taking advantage of the contact with the patients to offer screening to that needs it. Family medicine is the ideal framework for the activities of these

screenings "on hook," even the people who least motivated by prevention come to the family doctor when they feel ill (93% of the patients assigned to a family doctor visit the surgery a minimum of once every 5 years).

2. In family medicine, the predictive negative value — the probability that a certain disease is not the cause of the patient's problem — is more important than the predictive positive value, due to the low prevalence of disease versus the hospital context (where patients, select by family doctors, arrive). Thus, in family medicine, with a low prevalence of diseases, the positive predictive value of the test, decreases and will have more false (+) and less false (-). Consequently the family doctor must fish with a hook.

3. The family doctor should take individual decisions based on Bayesian probabilities — fishing with a hook rather than relying on the frequency probabilities offered by epidemiology and public health experts. The Bayesian approach makes things clearer. For example, if a study shows that in 100 smokers, 10 will develop lung cancer, a classical interpretation of the data can lead us think if I smoke I have a 10% probability of becoming ill. And this is not true. What the study really tells us is that the data (10 of every 100 smokers develop cancer) can be considered as a good starting point for making a prediction about the chances of developing cancer if I smoke. In contrast, a Bayesian approach would make it very clear that this is a highly incomplete knowledge, and, therefore, is not very useful without further information that raises the levels of certainty. Strictly speaking, for a Bayesian, it is incorrect to say, "I predict that there is a 10% chance of event P occurring — "lung cancer in smokers." Rather, he would say, "based on current knowledge, there is a 10% certainty that lung cancer will occur in smokers."

4. The family doctor has a different approach to statistical meanings — to fish with a net — and clinical meanings — to fish with a hook. If a statistical proof shows that a difference between the two measurements is significant at the 5% level ($p < 0.05$) it means that there is a 95% possibility that the difference found between treaties and controls is true and there is only a 5% possibility that the difference is due to random factors. Statistics is the method by which the effects of the chance are estimated. The statistical significance of some intervention does not always mean clinical significance and, vice versa, a non-statistically significant result can be considered significant in health. No matter how small "p" is, it does not speak of the magnitude of the differences or of clinical significance. Trivial differences may show "p" as statistically very significant if large numbers of subjects are studied. Thus the significance — the mathematical probability that the result did not occur by chance — is less relevant than the clinical significance — what the findings might mean if they were applied to a similar population.

5. The family doctor focuses on the effectiveness (fishing with a hook), compared to the efficacy (net fishing). The evaluation of the usefulness of health measures for the target population can be carried out by considering their effectiveness (actual conditions) and efficiency (laboratory conditions). Patients in clinical trials are selected to cooperate with the intervention being evaluated. But this does not happen with ordinary patients, so that they experience lower rates of success of the intervention that those reported in clinical trials.

The measure of efficiency tells us whether the treatment can work and provide more benefits than problems for those who are prescribed it under the restricted conditions of a study. Effectiveness tells us whether treatment has more advantages than disadvantages for those offered the treatment in ordinary life.

# References


Carreño Serra A. La estadística frecuentista y la estadística inferencial. El Teorema de Bayes. http://www.revistaseden.org/files/7-CAP%207.pdf.

Confucio. Los cuatro libros clásicos. Barcelona: Editorial S.A.; 1974.

http://www.amazon.co.uk/Cuadernos-medicina-familia-y-comunitaria/dp/8479781920.

http://www.elsevier.es/es/revistas/atencion-primaria-27/la-variabilidad-es-un-indicador-buena-gestion-13085349-reflexiones-medicina-familia-2006.

Leeflang MMG, Rutjes AWS, Reitsma JB, Hooft L, Bossuyt PMM. Variation of a test's sensitivity and specificity with disease prevalence. *CMAJ.* 2013, 185(11) E537.

Turabian Fernández JL, Pérez Franco B. Variablility is an Indicator of Good Clinical Management in Family Medicine. *Aten Primaria* 2006;37(3):160-166.

Turabian JL. Cuadernos de Medicina de Familia y Comunitaria. Una introducción a los principios de Medicina de Familia. Madrid: Díaz de Santos. 1995.

*Chapter 31*

# The Family Doctor as a Cubist or Abstract Painter

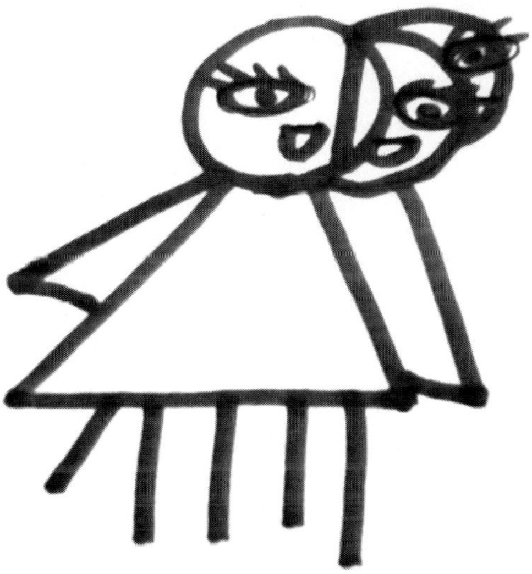

The cubist and abstract artists were constantly searching for the fundamental laws of painting, for new languages, and to open up new artistic perspectives. The difference between cubism and the more traditional painters is that cubism is not an art of imitation but of conception, which tends to rise the creation.

The search for new approaches, to invent rather than to imitate, is a characteristic of both cubism and family medicine — to convert a part into a whole, to produce an absolute reality from a fragmented reality. Cubists and abstract artists, such as family doctors, focus on translating a complex and individual reality, and on express the factors of the environment that are above the outer appearance. The abstract artists and family doctors try to go from the general to the particular. The family doctor goes from the general symptom of the patient to the particular symptom of that specific person and in that particular context.

The quest to learn more about reality led the creators of cubism to a view that held multiple perspectives in the search for a truly broad knowledge, and to a desire to transfer the weight and cohesion of the elements on the canvas.

To gather more information about a particular situation, the family doctor develops a broader and more complete vision of the facts. Usually, we see the data from a unique perspective: our perspective. But there is also a "cubist" vision. Looking for this broader view, we maintain the importance of our point of view but acknowledge that always it is possible to expand it to including the perspectives of others. This panoramic view is similar to that of the cubist painters: the analysis of an object seen after a succession of remarks and painted simultaneously from all possible points of views. All the elements included in a cubist picture help to expose a total image.

For the abstract artist and the family doctor the rupture between the perspective and conventional form (that had lasted since the Renaissance) is not intended to eliminate the form, but to emphasize its identity among other artistic elements. The space and the elements involved in it are an interrelated whole.

The perspectives of "cubists" or "abstract painters" in the management or treatment of uncertainty, or in the chaotic contexts where the family doctor works, are translated in "qualitative tools that are of assistance in taking decisions."

As in abstract art, in family medicine, an economy of means is sought: doing more with less. "The artist must economize in every detail," said Klee in 1909.

# References

Albers J. La interacción del color. Madrid: Alianza Forma; 1979.

De Torre G. Apollinaire y las teorías del cubismo. Barcelona: EDHASA; 1967.

Leigh H, Reiser MF. The patient. Biological, psychological, and social dimensions of medical practice. New York: Plenun Medical Book Company; 1992.

Paul Klee: Creative Confession and other writings. London: Tate Publishing, 2013.

Portera A. El espacio y el tiempo en el cubismo. JANO 2002; 63(1454): 10.

Rashomon. Wikipedia. [homepage on the Internet]. https://en.wikipedia.org/wiki/Rashomon.

Schmeller A. El cubismo. México: Editorial Hermes S.A.; 1959.

Tounier P. The meaning of persons. Reflections on a Psychiatrist's Casebook. London: SCM Press Ltd; 1963.

Undén A-L, Elofsson S. Health from the patient's point of view. How does it relate to the physician's judgement? Fam Pract 2001;18(2): 174-180. http://fampra.oxfordjournals.org/content/18/2/174.abstract?maxtoshow=&HITS=10&hits=10&RESULTFORMAT=&title abstract=Health+from+the+patient%2527s+point+of+view&searchid=QID_NOT_SET&stored_search=&FIRSTINDEX=0&fdate=1/1/2001&journalcode=fampract.

Chapter 32

# The Family Doctor as a Rhizome

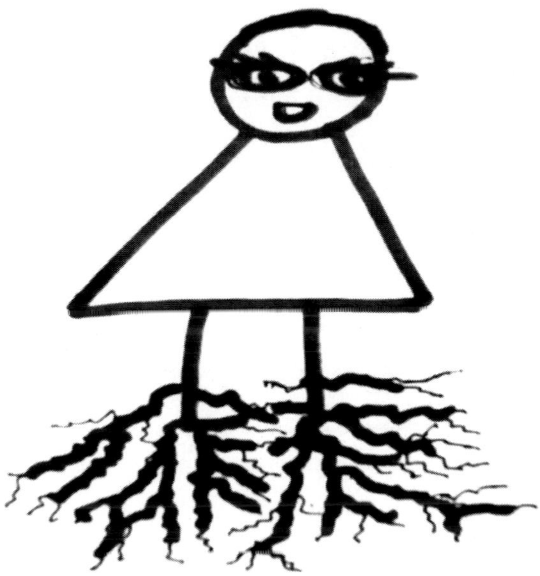

The "rhizome" is the underground portion of a generally horizontal interweaving of the roots of certain plants. The rhizome branches out and allows a portion of its network can develop other stems, thus stimulating the vegetative propagation of the plant, and its proliferation, sometimes very quickly. It is a system of vegetative reproduction in many plants, such as achimenes, canna, zantedeschia, lily, etc.

A first use of this metaphor is attributed to Carl Jung, the disciple of Freud: "Life always seemed to be like a plant that draws its vitality from its rhizome, the actual life of this plant is not as visible, it lies in its rhizome. What becomes visible above ground does not hold but a single summer, and then it withers (...). What we see is the flowering — and it disappears — but the rhizome remains."

Contemporary knowledge is marked by excessive compartmentalization and family medicine proposes its improvement, taking as a basis a new paradigm for the understanding of knowledge: the rhizome and transversality. The concept of transversality has a geometric origin and it means that which is opposite to the longitudinal, that is, to the length defined as the measured distance between two points. We could say that mainstreaming is something that fails to mark or define an area. Transversality is characterized by moving in several different areas without being at all influenced by the identity of each.

The rhizome is a descriptive model in which the organization of the elements does not follow a specific structure — with a base or root giving rise to multiple branches as in the familiar model of the tree — but where any element can affect or influence any other. In the rhizome, as in family medicine, the knowledge structure is not derived by logical means via a set of first principles, but is made simultaneously from all points under the reciprocal influence of the various observations and conceptualizations. This does not necessarily make a rhyzomatic structure labile. In one rhizome there are lines of solidity and organization determined by groups or sets of related concepts. These sets of concepts define relatively stable territories within the rhizome.

For the family physician, rather than taking a patient history, the analysis should be a geography: which lines are locked in a dead end or dead, which lines are active or alive, and which lines escape us and pull us?

What is hypertension or diabetes mellitus? What is white or black? What is proletarian or bourgeois? What is singular or plural? What is beyond the dualism (the multiplicity) that is not defined by the number of its term: is it not the elements or the sets that define the multiplicity? What defines it is the conjunction “Y.” Although there are only two terms, if there is a “Y” among them, it is neither one nor the other, but through the two, dragging them both in a non-parallel evolution.

Family medicine therefore uses the rhizome method in clinical management.

## References

Deleuze G, Guattari F. El anti-Edipo: capitalismo y esquizofrenia. Barcelona, Paidós Ibérica; 1985.

Deleuze G, Guattari F. Mil mesetas. Capitalismo y esquizofrenia. Valencia, Pre-textos, 1994.

Jung C. Recuerdos, sueños y pensamientos. Barcelona: Seix Barral; 2001.

Puig A. Sociología de las formas. Barcelona, Gustavo Gili, 1979.

*Chapter 33*

# The Family Doctor as Rouen Cathedral Painted by Monet

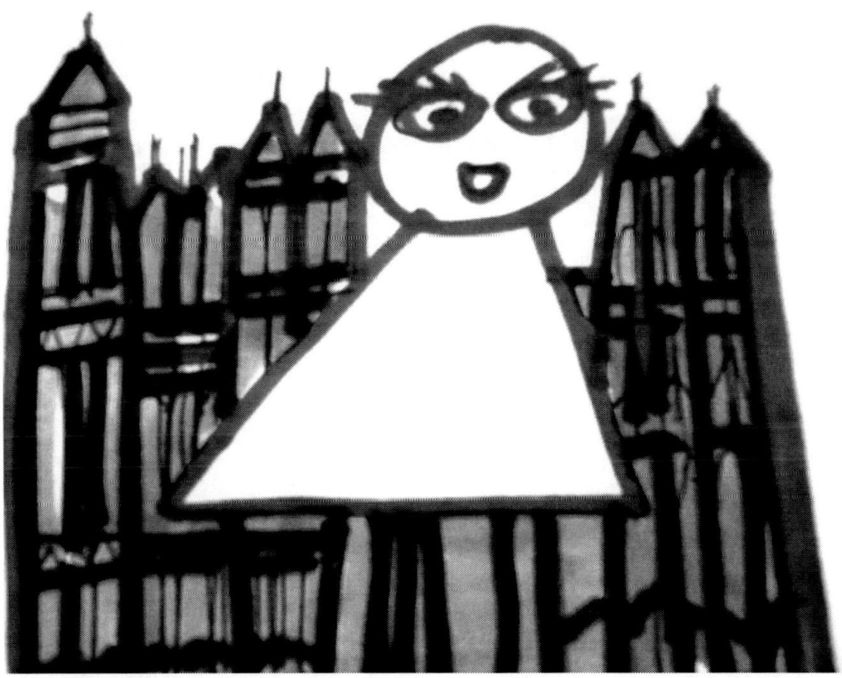

Why do leaves change colour in autumn? The leaves lose their lively green but flourish in wonderful colours. Finally, the leaves are gone. But before they change color and amaze us for weeks, after they crunch underfoot ... a wet layer of leaves protects new shoots until spring, and enriches the humus. The changing colours are like the colour of the stones of the city of Bologna that change over time.

Monet's paintings of Rouen Cathedral — a series of 31 views of the cathedral painted between 1892 and 1894 —show the front of the gothic cathedral of Rouen in different lighting conditions and climates. They represent a pictorial motif at different times to observe the changes resulting from the changes in natural light.

The family doctor sees the natural history of disease. This is basically a description of nature and is often perceived as a biological objective base on which to build or modify theory. In medicine, a major objective of the study it to reveal knowledge of the natural history of the disease — the natural story — because ignorance of this evolution can lead to significant errors of judgment in the therapeutic indications and prognosis.

Monet, in some sense, "despised" the architecture of the cathedral that had lost its grandeur. When he paints the cathedral from a position that is too close there is a near absence of perspective and the cathedral is dissected by towers and pinnacles. The building has become nothing more than a background, an excuse to show the real purpose of the composition: the ability of painting to represent the dynamic quality of light and atmosphere that is able to give life to something as stony and inanimate as the imposing facade of the gothic cathedral.

Like Monet, the family doctor focuses more on the natural history over time, but from the view of a single day. Thus, interpersonal and family continuity are of particular interest to family medicine. In ideal cases, this longitudinal relationship becomes a strong bond between the doctor and the patient-family, and is characterized by trust, loyalty and a sense of responsibility.

The family doctor retains a considerable amount of bio-psychosocial data on the patients that is set deep in doctor-patient relationship, and he uses this knowledge of human relations in his medical work. The continuity of care between the doctor and the patient builds trust and allows the doctor to use the available time more productively. Relational continuity improves the doctor-patient relationship.

For the family doctor, knowledge of the repetition of a certain pattern of expression of a symptom in a patient, or the disappearance of this predictable pattern, provides the diagnosis.

The accumulation of knowledge about the disease and the ways in which men respond to it, can be seen in family medicine, but requires an effort of observation and the maintenance of good records kept for years. It is as if the same observer in a village had carefully noted the dates of the appearance and fall of leaves, flowers, and the output of fruit ripening over a hundred species of cultivated and wild plants, the first dates each year when the swallows, swifts, and different species of butterflies appear, or when the first songs of the nightingales, cuckoos, and quail are heard.

## References

Ackerman D. Una historia natural de los sentidos. Barcelona: Anagrama S.A.; 1992.

Hjortdahl P, Borchgrevink CF. Continuity of care: influence of general practitioners' knowledge about their patients on use of resources in consultations. *BMJ.* 1991;303:1181–1184. http://www.ncbi.nlm.nih.gov/pmc/articles/PMC1671517/

Leigh H. Biopsychosocial approaches in primary care. State of the art and challenges for the 21st century. New York: Plenum Press; 1997.

Morrell D. The art of general practice. Oxford: Oxford University Press; 1991.

Santucci A. Il colore del tempo. Muri, intonaci e mattoni della Bologna antica e di quella presente. Bologna: Centro Editoriale S. Stefano s.r.l.; 2000.

*Chapter 34*

# The Family Doctor as a Detective

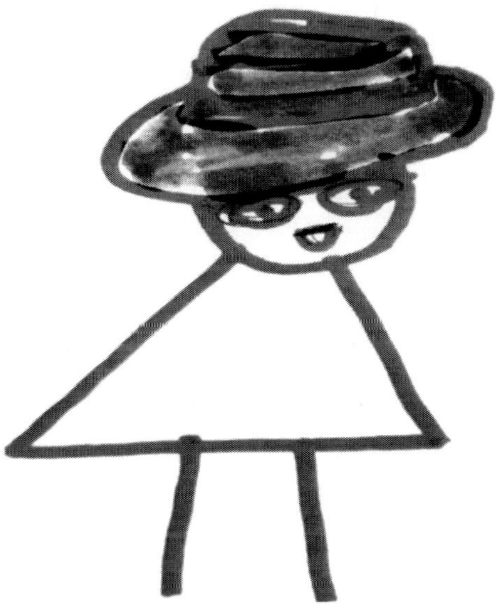

When a patient attends a consultation, the usual questions in the mind of the doctor are: "Where is the disease located?" and "What is the cause?" These questions are similar to those of a detective at a crime scene.

The family doctor is looking for a diagnosis of both the psychological and the physical aspects — a "whole" bio-psychosocial diagnosis. The natural way to reach this overall diagnosis seems to be by asking the patient lots of questions; as the detective. But he does not do it so; the detective does "many questions," but just the essential questions to clarify the case.

Detective work uses the same working model as the doctor. Sherlock and the family doctor use the same model: the scientific method. The need for evidence sits alongside the concept of the scientific method. The details hold the key to accessing a deeper reality that is inaccessible by other methods. For the detective Sherlock Holmes, clues or evidence at the crime scene can be found in the detail. In contrast to the police at Scotland Yard, Sherlock questions the details at the scene rather than asking questions.

Sherlock processes the information a very similar way to that of the family doctor. The doctor applies rationality to solve the problems of everyday life. The production of knowledge is achieved through logic and reason. Knowledge is divided by the detective in two parts:

1. Technical knowledge consisting of ordering and systematizing the experience. This is associated with generality.
2. Knowledge that has to do with time and practice. This is connected to resolving individual cases.

It is the production of knowledge and its systematization that can guide observations beyond what is visible. That is, after the logical ordering of information it possible to extract all the hidden information.

Another point to consider is the similarity between crime and disease. Both establish the identity of the subject behind every act through the network of observations and insignificant events that lead to the construction of the "other scene." To the detective the truth is extracted rather than found. The paradigm of clues (signs, symptoms) is linked with the idea of a hypothetical knowledge understood as the deciphering of various kinds of signs, from symptoms to writing. The sign must be understood as a footprint or mark. To move from seemingly insignificant facts to an unobservable complex reality it is necessary to put together a narrative.

Each crime (as in each disease) has a crime scene that can be carefully examined for clues. However, in many cases the evidence being analyzed is not a bloodstain or a carpet fibre but a set of relationships, a trend that has continued for years, emotions that are expressed suddenly or slowly, a personal experience of pathology.

The family doctor, like the detective in the case of a crime, is already committed and must preserve and analyze the evidence that has been gathered. The doctor must collect evidence, analyze traces, and as in the case of an investigation into a crime, both the detective and the doctor perform surveillance — for the doctor this may entail referring the patient for further consultations, new tests, and so on.

The detective and the doctor seek to re-order of a world that is in ruins. These repairs are performed by exposing the criminal who violated the law (the disease). This process of unveiling the truth locates the reasons (causes) of the health problem. These reasons can identify the pathology as well as the motives for the crime: revenge, anger, ambition or personal differences.

To explain the evidence from a holistic perspective requires the abilities of the detective and the doctor.

## References

Camilleri A. La voz del violín. Barcelona: Ediciones Salamandra, 2002.

http://apps.elsevier.es/watermark/ctl_servlet?_f=10&pident_articulo=90443461&pident_usuario=0&pcontactid=&pident_revista=27&ty=22&accion=L&origen=zonadelectura&web=www.elsevier.es&lan=es&fichero=27v47n09a90443461pdf001.pdf.

Le Fanu J. The case of the missing data. *BMJ* 2002;325:1490. http://bmj.com/cgi/content/full/325/7378/1490?etoc.

Pessoa F. El banquero anarquista y otros cuentos de raciocinio. Madrid: Alianza Editorial S.A.; 1986.

Roueché B. The Medical Detectives. New York: Washington Square Press; 1982.

Turabián JL, Samarín-Ocampo E, Minier L, Pérez-Franco B. Learning concepts of diagnosis in family medicine: the ''mark Robinson sign'' – the traces that should not be there. Aten Primaria. 2015; 47(9): 596-602. http://www.elsevier.es/ct-revista-atencion-primaria-27-articulo-aprendiendo-conceptos-del-diagnostico-medicina-90443461.

*Chapter 35*

# The Family Doctor as a Flying Kite

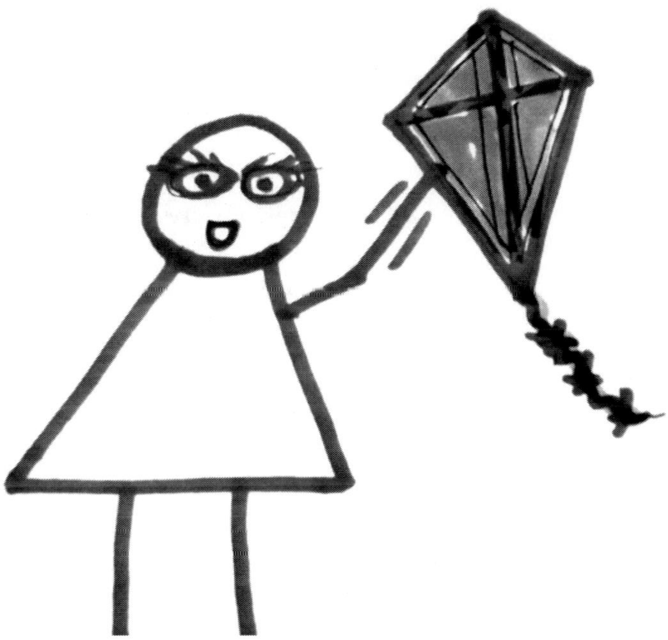

A kite is a very light plane, framed and covered or lined with cloth or paper and attached to a long string that is thrown into the air so that the air currents rise and move. The kite is the image of "freedom" flying in the air. The family doctor should learn to fly kites.

The kite flies because it is attached: if a kite is caught and thrown into the air without this it does not fly. However, if it is tied, the rope provides resistance against wind and kite flies. This is a very important principle for the family doctor.

The core of family medicine is empathy, in the sense of being able to identify, with imagination, the subjective experience of the patient to give a genuine validation and recognition of the experience. Empathy is the ability to perceive and understand the feelings of another person. With regard to communication, the other most important aspect is assertiveness, which is to defend one's position without feeling being aggressive. Assertive behavior involves retaining your legitimate rights without violating the rights of others.

Patients have to feel that the doctor respected their opinions. Even in situations of uncertainty, the family doctor should convey a sense of security and show that their opinions are significant. Empathy and assertiveness are related like the two axes X and Y. When there is a lot of empathy the family doctor should respond with a great deal of assertiveness; when there is little empathy, there should be little assertiveness.

The issue of rules and freedom in the office of family medicine is like flying a kite: It flies because it has a limit, it has freedom because it has limits. The family doctor should not get into the patient's skin (empathy), but for the patient to "fly" it is necessary that the family doctor demonstrates an assertiveness that is proportional to the circumstances.

## References

Confucio. Los cuatro libros clásicos. Barcelona: Editorial S.A.; 1974.

Derksen F, Bensing J, Kuiper S, van Meerendonk M, Lagro-Janssen A. Empathy: what does it mean for GPs? A qualitative study. Fam. Pract. 2015 32: 94-100. http://fampra.oxfordjournals.org/content/32/1/94.abstract.

Fuster V, Sampedro JL. La ciencia y la vida. Barcelona: Ramdom House Mondadori, S.A. P.; 2008.

Heath I. The mistery of general practice John Fry Trust Fellowship; 1995. http://www.nuffieldtrust.org.uk/sites/files/nuffield/publication/The_Mystery_of_General_Practice.pdf.

Ohm F, Vogel D, Sehner S, Wijnen-Meijer M, Harendza S. Details acquired from medical history and patients' experience of empathy – two sides of the same coin. BMC Medical Education 2013, 13:67. http://www.biomedcentral.com/1472-6920/13/67.

Rogers CR. A way of being. New York: Houghton Mifflin Company; 1995.

*Chapter 36*

# The Family Doctor as a Conductor

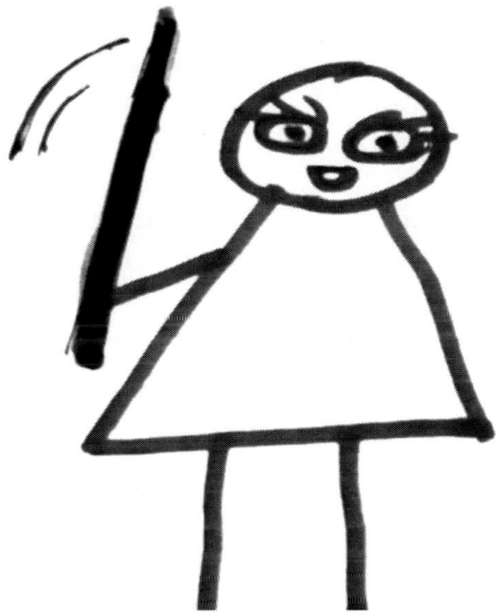

The conductor is the person who, in an orchestral context, in responsible for coordinating the different instruments.

His release coincides with the call symphonic music. The simple composition which is subordinate to a dominant simple form, is what we call a melodic composition. The complex composition is made up of several shapes that are subordinate to a main form. To us it can be very difficult to find the main form that gives the sound its great force. This musical composition is that we call a complex or symphonic composition. The complexity of polyphony and the Wagnerian drama, with its huge demands, contributed to the birth of the conductors. The conductor is therefore required for complexity.

The conductor is the figure of reference for the musicians of the orchestra. The conductor must coordinate the work of the musicians and the sounds of the instruments, and is also responsible for indicating the time and speed at which the musicians have to play: whether or not the music should be loud, and also the entrance of each group of instruments or soloists. The conductor is in charge of choosing the repertoire he thinks is most appropriate for each concert and must make every effort to tune the orchestra. If the orchestra is out of tune, the listener will be distracted and a great composition will be destroyed.

The sub-specialists of the orchestra are busy with sophisticated technology. But in fact, they work with the "simple." Besides, technological procedures monopolize the activity of the sub-specialist and they can result in you losing the holistic view of the patient. The sophisticated technology will not provide complete satisfaction for the patient, even when it performs well. Nobody heard the patients' doubts; nobody explored their feelings of depression, and while the artery was wide open, there remains the fear that the patient may die of a heart attack.

The study of the patient was fragmented. First, came the invasive cardiologist, after this, the non-invasive cardiologist, then the nuclear medicine specialist, and, finally, the cardiovascular surgeon. Each explained their technological approach. The patient could hear different comments that originated him more uncertainty. The procedure lacked a conductor to direct all these instruments.

The family physician works with the complex, and must be the reference figure for all others health system specialists. The family doctor, as the conductor, must coordinate the work of different medical and nursing professionals and arrange for medical interventions to be carried out in the proper sequence. The family doctor is in charge of choosing the repertoire of diagnostic tests and the therapeutic interventions he thinks are most appropriate for each case — leading the patient to the appropriate specialist and monitoring and reforming the activities of the specialists as he sees fit. That is, the family doctor as the conductor is responsible for coordinating all team members so that they retain a certain rhythm, and if he perceives an error, he corrects it.

The interventions of the family physician, in the role of conductor, must be comprehensive and involve actions that connect people, results, ideas, tasks, and powers, in context.

Therefore, the conductor in the health sector is the family doctor. He is the doctor who helps the patient to dispel fears, who integrates all patient studies, and who has the patience to solve all the patient's concerns.

# References

Kandinsky. De lo espiritual en el arte. Barcelona: Barral Editores, S. A.; 1982.

Gutierrez Jaramillo J. El médico de cabecera, una necesidad sentida. http://www.monografias.com/trabajos905/medico-cabecera-necesidad/medico-cabecera-necesidad2.shtml.

Pérez Franco B, Turabián Fernández JL. Framework of Competences of Family Doctors:Clinics or People? Aten Primaria 2007;39(1):41-3. http://www.elsevier.es/es-revista-atencion-primaria-27-articulo-marco-competencial-los-medicos-familia-13098264.

Turabian JL, Perez Franco B. The Doctor With Three Heads. Aten Primaria 2006;38(10): 570-3. http://www.elsevier.es/es/revistas/atencion-primaria-27/el-medico-tres-cabezas-13095929-reflexiones-medicina-familia-2006.

Chapter 37

# The Family Doctor as a Hiker in the Labyrinth

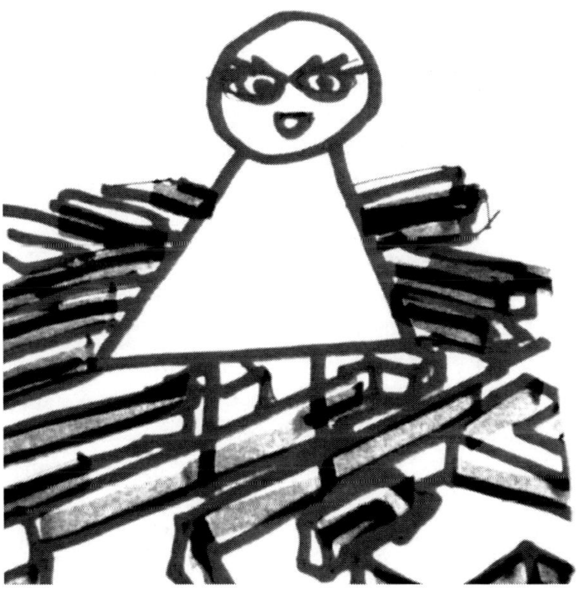

The image of the labyrinth can symbolize a religious man's journey throughout life, the allegorical figure on the "road to Jerusalem" that Christ walked on his last day and can be found on the floors of some medieval churches.

In Greek mythology, a well-known is that of Theseus and the Minotaur's labyrinth. Theseus was the son of Aegeus, King of Athens, and Etra. Aegeus had killed the son of Minos, so Creta did the war to Athens, which was quickly ravaged by famine and disease, and so Aegeus had to accept the conditions of Minos. The city of Athens was to deliver an annual tribute to Minos, the King of Crete. The city was required deliver each year 14 young people of the noblest families of the city, seven girls and seven boys. They were to be delivered to the Minotaur who was in the maze of the city. Theseus, decided to offer himself as tribute.

Ariadne, Minos's daughter fell in love with Theseus and she decided to help him because even if he successfully killed the Minotaur, getting out of the maze was impossible.

Therefore, she handed him a ball of gold thread. When he entered the labyrinth Theseus unrolling the ball and then found the exit. After killing the Minotaur, he followed the gold thread, which had been given to him by his beloved, to find the exit.

Each visit to the family doctor is like entering a labyrinth, a place formed by streets and crossroads. According to the dominant medical model, labyrinths have only one road. Decisions are made using a decision tree and algorithms: one starts by following a branch and when coming to a fork choose which of the two branches to take. On reaching another fork, one chooses again, and so on until reaching a branch that ends with a diagnosis. In this type of layout we know that at some point we will go to the center or out of the maze without making election; you just have to be patient and follow the algorithm.

But in real life each case has a multiple paths to the maze: a maze in which you can become lost. These mazes do not have a single path (or two inevitably connected routes) and the decisions taken at the forks determine whether or not the target is reached. This is the path where choices must be made between different ways and our choices may not lead us to the destination or even lead us to dead streets (dead ends), "islands," or sections of the route within the maze that are not connected to the perimeter, and that might result in circling over the same path in a continuous loop.

Moreover, in real life consultation in family medicine the roads are not always alternatives, may have different gateways, ramifications without end, and several equally valid exit doors, which are taken at one point in the query or set of queries in an arbitrary manner; the consultation ends, although it may continue in subsequent meetings with the same problem; without end. Many of the roads or medical interventions can have both positive and negative outcomes.

The concept of evidence-based medicine is too reductionist and biomedical and may be inappropriate for reducing the complexity of medical problems. A diagnosis can be simple, according to a conventional biomechanical pattern, but in family medicine, the diagnosis process is often imprecise and evolving. The diagnoses in family medicine are sometimes made forward, sometimes backward; sometimes you cannot make the diagnosis.

Also mazes are quintessentially English landscapes. The countryside is revealed in all its purity in the labyrinths. The maze is deliberately designed to be the longest route between A and B. It is the antidote to the everyday working life on the roads, which engineers designed in order to get from A to B in the shortest possible time. Here, the labyrinth is a spiritual quest.

The labyrinth, with one road leading from the entrance to the finish at its center, is a symbol of the deep spiritual quest of man, and has been one of the most lasting images of humanity for 4,000 years. For most of this time the classic maze has been formed by a pattern of seven rings. It was carved in the rocky walls of cliffs surrounded by water to define the sides of the roads and stones and grass clippings have created different lawn mazes. Intersections and decision-making points characterize labyrinths that go back about 400 years. By contrast, although it may seem contradictory, labyrinths do not pose the challenge of a puzzle, but rather the fascination of an allegorical journey, a rite of passage.

The family doctor deals each query (labyrinth) in a similar way to Theseus, equipped with a ball of gold thread (the bio-psychosocial vision), walking to an exit of the maze in a natural way that leads to unravelling facts and re-stating the problem in a way that open up a solution for treatment. But the family doctor walks the labyrinth of his professional life as a spiritual journey, fascinated by what he sees on this long road, day after day.

## References

Spielthenner G. The principle of double effect as a guide for medical decision-making. *Med Health Care and Philos* 2008; 11: 465-473.

http://springer.r.delivery.net/r/r?2.1.Ee.2Tp.XARIh.BxR8%2ag..T.GZrE.35gK.DSZMEYL0.

Coderre S, Wright B, McLaughlin K. To think is good: querying an initial hypothesis reduces diagnostic error in medical students. *Acad Med* 2010 Jul;85(7):1125-9. http://www.ncbi.nlm.nih.gov/pubmed/20592507.

Sweeney K. How can evidence-based medicine help patients in general practice? *Fam Pract* 1996; 13(6): 489-490. http://fampra.oxfordjournals.org/content/13/6/489.full.pdf.

Fisher A. Mazes and follies. Norwich: Jarrold Publishing; 2004.

Turabian JL. Helping "Dr. Theseus" leave the labyrinth of multiple drug interactions. *BMJ* 2015;350:h1059. http://www.bmj.com/content/350/bmj.h1059/rr-0.

Turabian JL. "Ariadne and the Miotaur." Qualitative tools to address multimorbidity in family medicine. *BMC Medicine* 2014, 12:223. http://www.biomedcentral.com/1741-7015/12/223/comments.

Turabián JL, Pérez Franco B. A way of helping ''Mr. Minotaur'' and ''Ms. Ariadne'' to exit from the multiple morbidity labyrinth: The ''master problems''. Semergen. 2016; 42 (1): 38-48. http://www.elsevier.es/es-revista-semergen-medicina-familia-40-articulo-un-modo-ayudar-al-sr--90447188.

Horace Walpole. Ensayo sobre la jardineria moderna. Editorial Jose J. de Olañeta, 2003.

*Chapter 38*

# The Family Doctor as a Lawyer

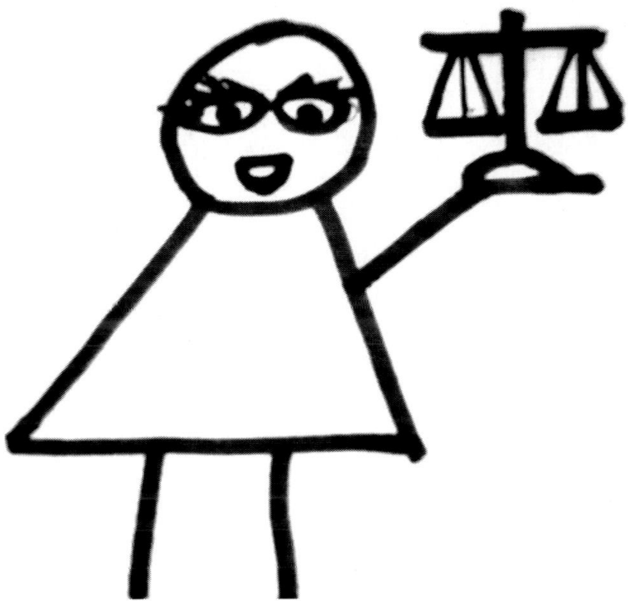

The lawyer is an independent professional who, as a consultant and representative of a person, defends their rights and interests.

The lawyer is a versatile technician who, depending on their areas of expertise, can provide services defend a person's interests in all kinds of legal proceedings, negotiations, and drafting of all types of public and private contracts. They provide advice and brokering for all types of real estate transactions, tax advice, counseling and rights management, defence against sanctions, and so on.

The family doctor spends years serving the interests of their patients and relatives. He knows his strengths and weaknesses. Through these multiple inquiries the doctor has established bonds of affection and commitment, always seeking the best for the patient. Thus, the family doctor sees beyond the medical aspects. The family physician becomes an advocate for the patient and recommends solutions that are best for the patient. The family doctor looks for the best sub-specialist to help solve the complex problems of their patients.

In this way, the family doctor is the patient's advocate or social agent. Family physicians are engaged in their communities and can play the role of "patient advocate," encouraging the population to have access to health, social resources, health education, and to use these resources efficiently.

The specialist doctor who is not a family doctor tends to work differently from the attorney. For the physician, the patient "is guilty" (it does not matter to have a mistake and to call guilty or sick to a healthy patient, that is, from an epidemiological point of view, does not mind incurring a type I error: take for real a false positive; so giving more value to the test positive, although they may be false).

However, from point of view of the lawyer, the individual is innocent until proven otherwise (he prefers to err by calling "not guilty" instead to have a fault in reverse, that is, he prefers to incur the type II error: take as true a false negative).

From an epidemiology perspective, when the outcome of a clinical trial, or a diagnosed test is expressed in dichotomous terms (useful or not), there are four ways in which the conclusions could be related to reality.

| | REAL DIFFERENCE | | |
|---|---|---|---|
| CONCLUSION OF STATISTICAL TEST | | Present | Absent |
| | Statistical difference | CORRECT | INCORRECT (Error Type I or Alfa) (Comparable to false positive) |
| | No statistical difference | INCORRECT (Type II error or beta) (Comparable to false negative) | CORRECT |

Thus, examples for the type I error would be:

He believes that the patient is sick, even though in reality he is healthy.

He finds the defendant guilty, even though he is actually innocent.

For type II error:

He believes that the patient is healthy, although in reality he is sick.

He argues that the accused is not guilty, even though in actually he is guilty.

In his role as patient advocate, the family doctor has to fear to the error type I, instead the type II error. From an epidemiological point of view the family doctor has to be more of a lawyer than a medic.

## References

Barker DJP, Rose G. Epidemiology in medical practice. New York: Churchill Livingstone1984. -Fletcher RH, Fletcher SW, Wagner EH. Clinical epidemiology. The esssentials. Baltimore: Williams & Wilkins; 1982.

http://www.amazon.co.uk/Cuadernos-medicina-familia-y-comunitaria/dp/8479781920.

Last JM. The iceberg: "completing the clinical picture" in general practice. The Lancet 1963; 282 (7297): 28 - 31. http://www.lancet.com/journals/lancet/article/PIIS0140-6736(63)92546-7/fulltext.

Lilienfeld AM, Lilienfeld DE. Fundamentos de epidemiología. México: Addison-Wesley Iberoamericana; 1986.

Turabian JL. Cuadernos de Medicina de Familia y Comunitaria. Una introducción a los principios de Medicina de Familia. Madrid: Díaz de Santos. 1995.

*Chapter 39*

# The Family Doctor as an Ecologist

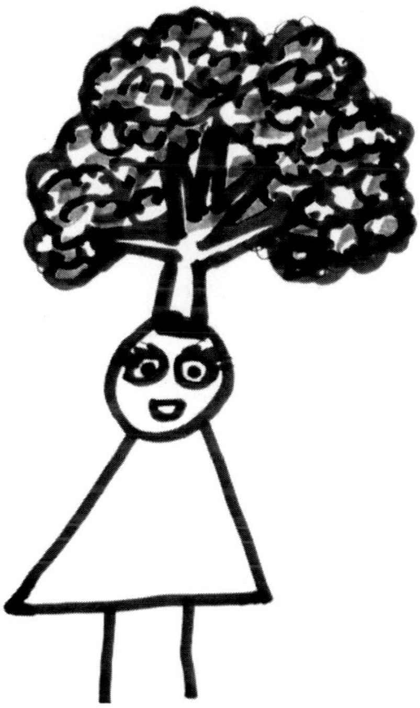

Ecology is the study of relationships that connect all members of a system — the study of the functional relationships between organisms and environments.

It is currently the case that specialization has become the only way to develop. Specialization and fragmentation is the inevitable result of the mechanistic approach to medicine where the body is divided into parts, chemically or surgically manipulated, or where defective parts are changed as if it were a machine. However, the real problem is the dysfunctional relationship between each element, and when medicine studies only the detail of parts of the body it loses the overall dynamics of life. Medical interventions have achieved success with the advance of biochemistry, but these only occur if we reduce the problem to a biochemical phenomenon and have a drug to deal with it.

As an environmentalist, the vision of the family doctor maintains that the whole is greater than the sum of its parts, and that individual symptoms should not be isolated but viewed as a pattern of disharmony in a system. The ecological approach to health suggests that the mind and body are not separate and that mental and emotional imbalances have physical effects, and vice versa. It also suggests that the individual cannot be isolated from their life circumstances.

In addition, the formula for survival lies not in power but in symbiosis. This is a process where different parties who see different aspects of a problem can constructively explore their differences and reach solutions that go beyond their own limited vision. An example is the lichens in the plant kingdom. In every corner of nature life is a collective enterprise. Progress is an increase of relations with the environment. Ecology is about networks. To understand living systems it is important to understand their relational networks. Living organisms are networks of living organisms. Living systems should be understood as networks of interacting systems.

We could draw a system schematically as a network with a few nodes. Each node represents an individual or organization, but if we expanded view, each organism appears as a network. That is, when expanded, each node in the connection network becomes a network, and so on. In other words, life consists of networks within networks. Although we tend to prioritize these networks as large or small, up or down, placing the minor in the majors, this is only a human projection. There really is no hierarchy, there are only networks nesting within other networks. Individuals themselves are networks of relationships located in larger networks.

In ecological thinking, the main thing is relationships; the borders of a certain object are secondary. Progress is achieved by increasing protection of the complexity of the individual against the contingency of environmental uncertainty. Every innovation that increases the degree of independence of a system from its environment is progressive for the system. The independence of a complex system within its environment is not achieved in isolation, but rather, with a sophisticated network of relationships between them. Progressive innovations were the "invention" of the feathers of birds that helped the birds to become independent of temperature changes and flying, free to live immersed in water, or to stand.

## References

Bonn D. Biocomplexity: look at the whole, not the parts. *Lancet* 2001; 357:288.

Dersu Uzala (1975 film). Wikipedia. [homepage on the Internet]. https://en.wikipedia.org/wiki/Dersu_Uzala_(1975_film).

Haggerty J, Burge F, Lévesque J-F, Gass D, Pineault R, Beaulieu M-D, Santor D. Operational Definitions of Attributes of Primary Health Care: Consensus Among Canadian Experts. Ann Fam Med. 2007; 5:336-344. http://www.annfammed.org/cgi/content/full/5/4/336.

March D, Susser E. The eco- in eco-epidemiology. *Int. J. Epidemiol.* 2006; 35: 1379-1383. http://ije.oxfordjournals.org/cgi/content/full/35/6/1379?etoc.

March D, Susser E. The eco- in eco-epidemiology. *Int. J. Epidemiol.* 2006 35: 1379-1383. http://ije.oxfordjournals.org/cgi/content/full/35/6/1379?etoc.

Turabián Fernández JL, Pérez Franco B. Fábulas Médicas: El Efecto Iceberg. Madrid: Marbán; 2013. http://libreriatecnicosleo.com/es/ciencias-medicas-y-naturales-/26863-jose-lis-turabian-fabulas-medicas-en-atencion-primaria-4-tomos.html.

Turabián Fernández JL, Pérez Franco B. Fábulas Médicas: El Efecto Mariposa. Madrid: Marbán; 2013. http://libreriatecnicosleo.com/es/ciencias-medicas-y-naturales-/26863-jose-luis-turabian-fabulas-medicas-en-atencion-primaria-4-tomos.html.

Turabián Fernández JL, Pérez Franco B. Fábulas Médicas: El Efecto Barnum. Madrid: Marbán; 2013. http://libreriatecnicosleo.com/es/ciencias-medicas-y-naturales-/26863-jose-luis-turabian-fabulas-medicas-en-atencion-primaria-4-tomos.html.

Turabián Fernández JL, Pérez Franco B. Fábulas Médicas: La Ley de Stevens. Madrid: Marbán; 2013. http://libreriatecnicosleo.com/es/ciencias-medicas-y-naturales-/26863-jose-luis-turabian-fabulas-medicas-en-atencion-primaria-4-tomos.html.

Turabian JL, Pérez Franco B. Actividades Comunitarias en Medicina de Familia y Atención Primaria. Madrid: Díaz de Santos; 2001. http://www.amazon.es/Actividades-comunitarias-medicina-atenci%C3%B3n-primaria/dp/8479784741.

Turabian JL, Perez Franco B. la disciplina mas ecológica es la medicina de familia. SIIC Salud. 2010. http://www.siicsalud.com/dato/arsiic.php/96635.

*Chapter 40*

# The Family Doctor as a Marathon Runner

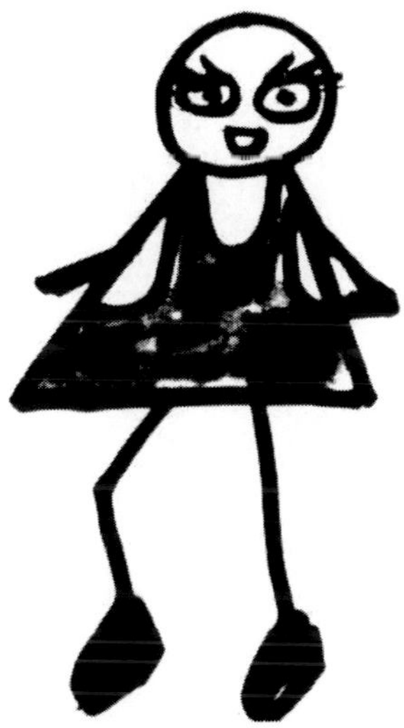

A marathon is a long distance race consisting of running a distance of 42 Km.

The origins of the marathon can be located in the myth of the heroic deeds of the Greek soldier, Philippides, who, in 490 BC, died of fatigue after running about 37 km from Marathon to Athens to announce victory over the Persian army.

Family doctors are like marathon runners. Do they have to run the Berlin, Boston, Chicago, London, New York or Tokyo marathon? Or all of them?!!?

The family doctor usually works from the same office, often over a long time, perhaps several years. The daily round of consultation is hard, and year after year it becomes even harder. More than being in great physical condition, the marathon runner and the family doctor need good psychological conditions. Technical training for the marathon runner can help him to achieve a good performance and favorable feelings on the day of the marathon. That same applies to the career and the clinical practice of the family doctor.

Continuity of care, perhaps over many years, is considered to be a defining characteristic of family medicine and an essential attribute of primary care in both developed and emerging countries. Yet, although many positive factors of this interpersonal continuity have been described, there are also areas of uncertainty and negative risk. The relationship established between a doctor and a patient during the disease process is extremely important. This rich and complex relationship influences the course of disease and treatment efficacy and itself has a curative value.

To serve the same patients over time is complex and difficult. How can the family doctor reach a certain pace to ensure that he does not go "too slow" or "too fast"? The answer lies in the objective that we have. Both the family physician and the marathon runner must know his mental capacity to meet the challenge of the marathon (concentration, sacrifice, frustration tolerance, self-confidence), to retain it along the course of 42 km — or in the case of the professional life of the family doctor, across 200,000, 300,000 or more queries. The ability to concentrate enables us to face the last kilometres of the marathon, and we are able (or not) to reach that goal and enjoy (or not) the end of the race. So, if we have a slip, a fall, a pain, a sense of discouragement, etc., we may lose concentration during the race, and this may prevent us from continuing in the race.

The family physician and the marathon runner need to have confidence. If at the beginning of the race we are absolutely sure that we are ready to finish it according to what we have proposed, we are unlikely to get carried away by feelings of fear, anxiety, despair or concern and, therefore, it is easier to keep within our scheduled time.

Similarly, the family physician and marathon runner, must think in advance about the difficulties. It may be this the most important element to have a good concentration during the marathon. In fact, the more we can control the race circumstances, the less likely we are to be surprised by events that alter our style of race and, therefore, divert our concentration.

Are you ready to run the marathon for 35 or 40 years of seeing patients in the service of family medicine?

# References

Ogur B, Hirsh D. Learning through longitudinal patient care-narratives from the Harvard Medical School-Cambridge Integrated Clerkship. *Acad Med* 2009; 84(7):844-50. http://journals.lww.com/academicmedicine/pages/articleviewer.aspx?year=2009&issue=07000&article=00011&type=abstract.

Rafferty G, Mills J. The vet. Beyond the surgery door. London: BBC Books; 1989.

Roth W-M. Auto/biography as Method: Dialectical Sociology of Everyday Life. Review Essay: Zdenek Konopásek (Ed.) (2000). Our Lives as Database—Doing a Sociology of Ourselves: Czech Social Transitions in Autobiographical Research Dialogue. *Forum Qual Soc Res,* 3(4): 17. http://www.qualitative-research.net/fqs-texte/4-02/4-02review-roth-e.htm.

Turabián Fernández JL, Pérez Franco B. "Observaciones, intuiciones y anécdotas, desde la perspectiva del médico, para una teoría de la historia natural de la continuidad interpersonal. Los colores del tiempo." *Rev Clin Med Fam.* 2015; 8 (2). http://www.revclinmedfam.com/articulo.php?art=412.

*Chapter 41*

# The Family Doctor as an Archaeologist

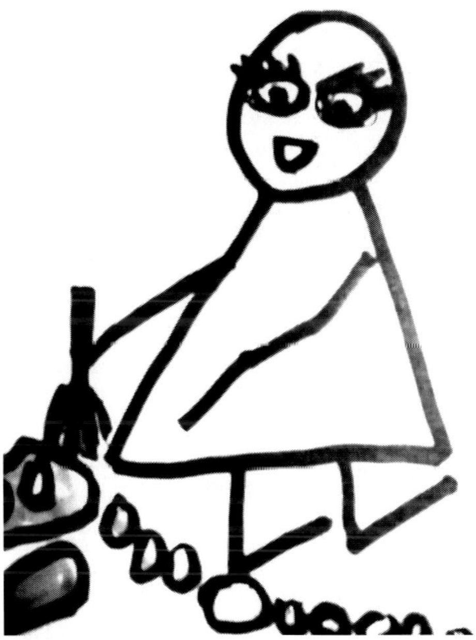

Archaeologists are responsible for studying the human past through the remains and materials left by the people who have inhabited the earth. Their job is to locate, document, analyze and preserve the remains of other cultures and then disseminate the results of that investigation. They study the human past through remains such as bones, textiles, ceramics, tools, landscape features and buildings. They engage in digging, identifying, recording and preserving these remains. This work also involves laboratory analysis, research, asset management and planning advice. These researchers perform their work in a systematic, unhurried and meticulous manner. It is a job that requires planning and method.

Performing a clinical history of a patient in family medicine and developing a related "problem list" forces doctors to locate, document, analyze, identify and record ancient remains. The medical history and list of problems in family medicine are like archaeological relics from the past: vestiges that remain in the ground, from small devices or ceramics, bones, coins, shells, snails, beetles fragments, seeds, pollen ... to large Gothic cathedrals, documents and paintings. There are often abundant traces!

The "excavations" — both archaeological and clinical — give rise to an enormous amount of data. This information provides an excellent aid to understanding the past and the present, but all the data is immense and interpretation needs to be based on only a selection. Quantitative analysis (theoretically "objective") of this multitude of data can be like "the mountain that gives birth to a tiny mouse." Perhaps one could think of a computer system, or electronic medical records, summarizing or prioritizing data, as in the case of multi-morbidity. But prioritizing health problems according to the quantitative or mathematical analysis of all the material can be unhelpful and, to some extent a dangerous tool.

When carried out correctly, family medicine involves identifying the plethora of data and multi-morbidity and using clinical judgment to decide when to treat, and to what extent. From time immemorial, health professionals know that the information obtained from a patient will be different depending on where the focus is placed. Reducing the heterogeneity and complexity of the plethora of information and multi-morbidity can theoretically be achieved in various ways.

Family doctors have to know "where to dig," and so their preparation and intuition are fundamental. The findings are the result of a systematic search in a territory that is thought to have been "populated in ancient times" and in this case, the results of a series of laborious techniques entailing complexity and cost, such as physical examinations, analytical complementary tests and imaging. Once the archaeologist has obtained a wealth of information from the previous phases of the research, like the family doctor, he has to "think to fit all the pieces." To do this, the information must be sorted, a critical study must be made, and contradictory data eliminated. Thus the findings are summarized and the case is diagnosed.

## References

Martlew R. Information Systems in Archaeology. Gloucester: New Standard Archaeology. Alan Sutton Publishing Limited; 1984.

Ray Hyatt. Collaboration between generalists in primary and secondary care is needed. BMJ 2012;345:e5148. http://www.bmj.com/content/345/bmj.e5148?etoc=).

Turabian Fernández JL, Perez Franco B. La historia clínica electrónica: ¿comer sopa con tenedor? Cuadernos de Gestión. 2204;10(4):175-188. http://es.scribd.com/doc/34257833 /hacp-electronica-sopa-con-tenedor-cuad-gestion-2004#scribd).

Turabian JL, Perez Franco B. Family medicine clinical sessions: they do exist! Aten Primaria. 2010;42(12):588-590. http://www.elsevier.es/es/revistas/atencion-primaria-27/sesiones-clinicas-medicina-familia-haberlas-haylas-13188677-editorial-2010).

*Chapter 42*

# The Family Doctor as a Kitchen Chef

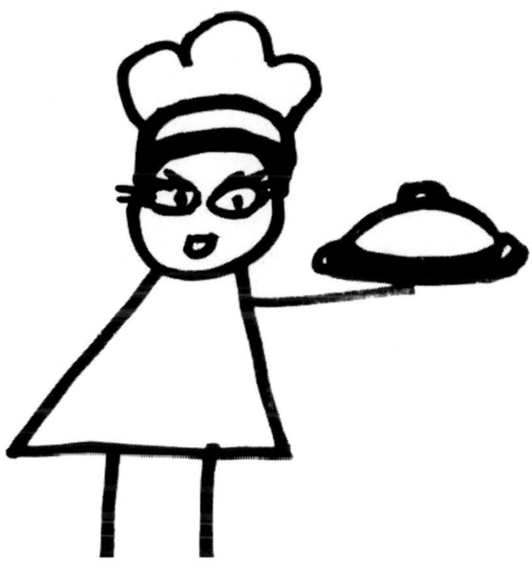

The chef, a word that originates in French, is the "organizer and coordinator of the work in the kitchen, and is responsible for the design of menus, for letters of suggestion and technical specifications, and establishes the price of the dishes." The chef takes care of the supply and quality of the dishes prepared by the kitchen team he leads. This concept is used in everyday language to designate the person whose profession or occupation is cooking.

So, A smorgasbord, a hot pot, a cocktail? How does the chef cook it? And the family doctor, how does he cook to his patients?, underdone?, well done?, cooked in its point?, cooked "al dente"? The "cooking" of patients is currently considering not only a necessity, but also an art. Today we also tend to differentiate between eating and feeding. Likewise, we must distinguish between cured with drugs or cure as a result of "unlocking scenarios."

The cook or chef is a kind of alchemist, who uses his power to conceal or mix food materials with the ultimate goal of reaching the joy or pleasure of dinner (flavors, emotions). "Cooking" requires the processing of foods to make them more pleasant; it is a process that occurs at a "micro" level: it is bubbling, fermenting; it is a chemical interaction, a nuclear fission. The process of cooking is the condition to allow for growth. It is the smallest unit of generative action for a person to come to new perceptions of the context and of itself.

The family doctor "cooks" by combining contrasting or conflicting ingredients: this is an interaction between people, between ideas, between contexts, between methods, between now and the future outlook, and with oneself (with our feelings, beliefs, symbols, language ...).

During the "cooking" new flavors, colors and textures are produced. During the "cooking" new ideas and perceptions, new connections, and new developments occur from any of the existing potential. During the "cooking" ideas and words interact leading to a qualitatively different state, and to greater organization.

Before entering the kitchen — the surgery of the family doctor — to see what we might prepare, it is good to have taken a look at the most common recipes, to know how much time we have, what ingredients we need, if we can go out to buy what is missing, if it is necessary to focus on these concepts, and the level of sophistication of the dish we intend to prepare. Having the ingredients on hand and in relative order of use really helps to control the kitchen space (and patient consultation).

Also keep in mind that a grumpy man can never become a master of culinary art since the disorder of his gastric juices destroys the peculiar excellence that should govern the palate: it is left stale and tasteless.

Bon appetite!

# References

Adler HM. The history of the present illness as treatment: who's listening, and why does it matter?. *J Am Board Fam Pract* 1997;10:28-35. http://www.jabfm.org/content/10/1/28.full.pdf.

Brody H. Placebo response, sustained partnership, and emotional resilience in practice. JABFP 1997;10:72-74. http://www.jabfm.org/content/10/1/72.full.pdf.

Cousins N. Anatomy of an illness as perceived by the patient. Reflections on healing and regeneration. New York: W.W. Norton & Company; 1979.

Elbow P. Writing without teachers. Oxford: Oxford University Press; 1998.

Enelow A, et al. *Interviewing & Patient Care*. New York: Oxford University Press, 1996.

Neighbourg R. The inner consultation. Lancaster: MTP press; 1991.

Pierce H. The Household Manager, 1863. En: Ben Schott. Miscelánea gastronómica de Schott. Barcelona: El Aleph Editores; 2005.

*Chapter 43*

# The Family Doctor as an Interpreter

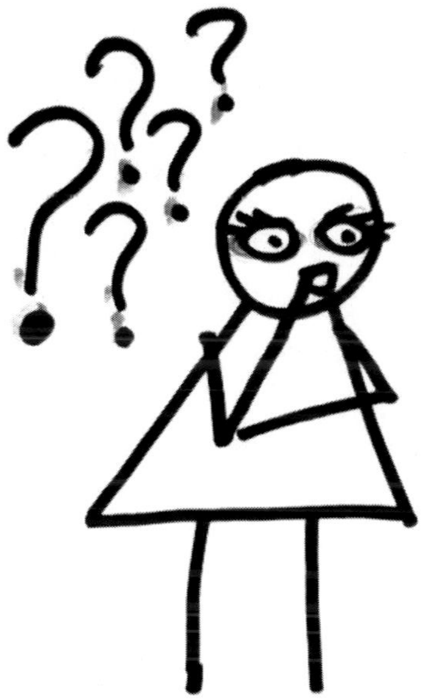

The word "interpreter" means mediator or intermediary. Therefore, the interpreter is a language professional that mediates between two or more people who do not speak the same language so that they can communicate.

We receive communications from human beings and from social system too. This is a system of meanings. The disease is a system of interpretation and to understand the disease we have to see a network of relations. The emotional response expressed by the patient has the effect of a linguistic transfer from social complexity to mental complexity.

The concept of "meanings" refers to the way in which human experience is organized. The patient experience is opened during the clinical consultation. The system generates meanings. The language spoken during the clinical encounter provides partial evidence of the meanings of the patient. The patient has a personal concept of disease, but this is only one of many interpretation systems that contribute to the knowledge of the person and the social awareness of the disease.

The work of the family doctor is to try to understand the meaning of the illness for the patient and to interpret it in medical terms. Likewise, the pathologist validates the clinical diagnosis; the patient validates the communication process. This requires the clinician to understand and respond to the concerns and feelings of the patient, and the relationship between disease and the patient's life. Every person (patient) is unique. Unlike what occurs in the old clinical method used by other specialists, which protects the professional from the patient and makes him a detached observer of the patient, the clinical method of the family doctor is open to expressions of feeling unwell (some of which can be annoying to the doctor).

The clinical encounter represents two distinct and separate worlds, one from the perspective of the doctor and another from the patient's experience. The family doctor needs to have an "interpreter" to translate these different languages. A common mistake, which can make a patient look to the family doctor like a "problem," is the doctor's lack of knowledge and understanding of he patient's interpretations from the perspective of their own culture.

The disease is expressed as a contrast rather than a separate and unambiguous entity, as a contrast between systems of relations. The family doctor has to share the patient's interpretative codes to achieve a minimally intelligible communication. When we raise opinions and undertake analysis without prior agreement with the patient on the codes of meaning, we run the risk of not knowing what we are talking about. How to be sure of interpreting well a look or a smile?

The family doctor makes interpretations, understands values and makes judgement from the start to the end of his work. From the point of view of the family doctor, patient care means interpretation. A medical history cannot be taken if the doctor fails to establish any contact with the minds of those with which he works.

If the discipline of clinical medicine is related to the discipline of the translator, then doctors should learn the working methods of the same.

# References

Bracken P, Thomas P. Time to move beyond the mind-body split, *BMJ* 2002;325 1433-1434. http://bmj.com/cgi/content/full/325/7378/1433?etoc.

Churchill Jr. CJ. Ethnography as Translation. *Qualitative Sociology*. 2005; 28 (1): 3 – 24.

La Salud Mental Relacional. Advances in relacional mental Health. *An International On-line Journal.* 2002; 1(1). http://www.bibliopsiquis.com/asmr/0101/0101editorial.htm.

Macchioli FA. Enrique Pichon-Rivière: la teoría de la enfermedad única a través de algunos de sus recorridos nosográficos. *ÁREA 3. CUADERNOS DE TEMAS GRUPALES E INSTITUCIONALES.* 2010; 14. http://www.area3.org.es/uploads/a3.14.teu.fmacchioli.pdf.

Rogers CR. On becoming a person. Boston: Houghton Mifflin Company; 1961.

Chapter 44

# The Family Doctor as a Gardener

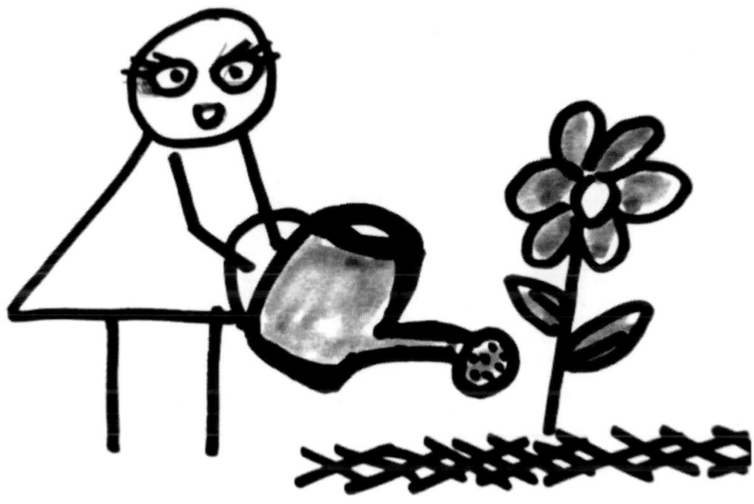

The gardener takes care of the gardens. He knows he may have to grow a variety of plants such as flowers, shrubs, trees and lawns.

It is important that the family doctor acts as if he were a gardener. Like the gardener, the family doctor serves very different patients. The gardener patiently listens and watches. Gardeners are sensitive to their plants and they pamper trees and plants,

In ancient times the dominant behavior of people resembled that of the warden whose primary mission was to preserve the balance, the manifestation of the "manifold wisdom of God." During the modern era, the dominant behavior became that of the gardeners, for there can be no order in the world if not through their work and efforts. For Bauman, gardeners are the most enthusiastic creators of utopias. However, the era of postmodernism is the time of the hunter who is not interested in the balance of things and in garden design; the hunter is only concerned with the task of hunting to fill his pouch.

When we plant a rose seed, we realize that it is small, but do not criticize it for that. We treat it as a seed, we water it. When we see the first shoots of the plant coming out of the ground, we not condemn them for being immature and undeveloped. We do not criticize the shoots because their cocoons came closed. We follow the process and care for the plant according to each stage of development. The rose is a rose from the time we plant the seed until it dies. Inside it is, at all times, achieving its full potential. It always seems to be in flux; every stage, at every moment, and it is fine as it is.

Family doctors can neglect the development of the innate potential of their patients. So, the doctor may give the patient excessive instructions ("You have to do such and such ..."). And, even worse, the doctor may criticize the patient for not having done what the doctor told them to do.

If the family doctor has the attitude of being the one who knows things, and the patient is the one who does not know things, he will try to quickly judge the patient. However, what the family doctor needs is to draw from the depths of his own experience to intuit where the patient is, and to helps him grow — to "encourage stems and blossom" ... Family doctors have to learn the craft of the gardener.

Similarly, the errors committed by the patient can be seen as an important part of their development. We learn from mistakes. There are no bad mistakes. The good gardener knows when the seed needs alkaline earth and when the seed needs acidic soil. The competent family physician should be able to help develop the style of the patient. The family doctor should know how and when to provide "water" for his patient, when to prepare the soil, to plant and to fertilize it. And for that, the first thing is to avoid the negative concepts that inhibit the development of innate learning process. As Walt Whitman said: "Do not let the day end without having grown a little," and: "I think a blade of grass is no less than the day of the stars."

## References

Bauman Z. tiempos liquidos. Barcelona: Tusquets Editores; 2007.
Cho Wang J. The Chinese Garden. Oxford: Oxford University Press; 1988.
Elbow P. Writing without teachers. Oxford: Oxford University Press; 1998.
Horace Walpole. Ensayo sobre la jardineria moderna. Editorial Jose J. de Olañeta, 2003.
Nakane K. Kyoto Gardens. Osaka: Hoikusha; 1979.
Saito K. Japanese gardens. Tokyo: Shufunotoma Co., Ltd; 1988.
Walt Whitman. Hojas de hierba. Madrid: Alianza Editorial; 2012.

*Chapter 45*

# The Family Doctor as a Journalist

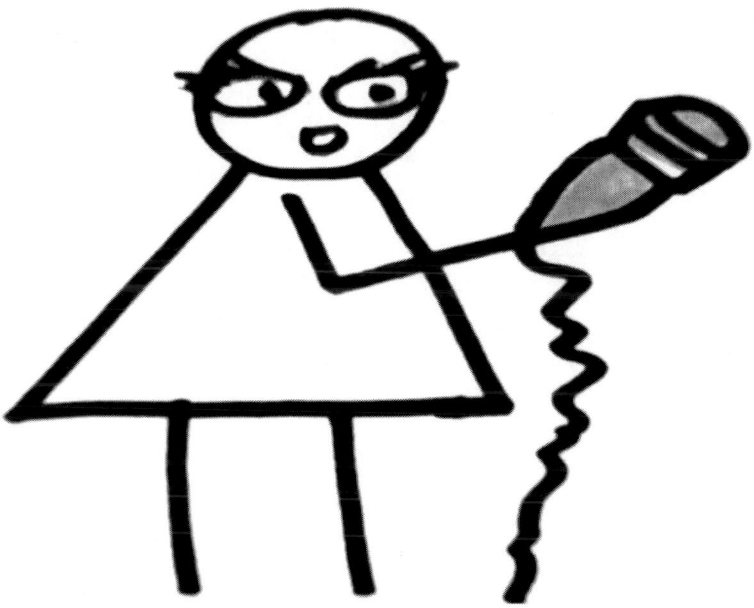

Imagine that you have the opportunity to interview your favourite character. You will be a journalist for a few minutes. This is the person you most want to get to know. Perhaps it's Louis Armstrong, Johnny Depp, Nicolas Cage, Mickey Mouse, Paul Gauguin, Cristobal Colon, Albert Einstein, Stalin, Julius Caesar, Karl Marx, Alexander the Great, Aristotle, Abraham Lincoln, William Shakespeare, Mohammed, Napoleon Bonaparte, or Jesus. You will have to focus your full attention, listening only to the character without regard to anything else. What questions will ask him?

Listening sounds easy, but it is the most complex and difficult medical tool in the doctor's repertoire. Listening is not a passive task. It is about "hearing problems that are not verbalized, and assist the patient without talking." Effective communication depends much more on our ability to be good listeners than it does on the ability to say things to the patient. Most doctors mistakenly believe that they listen more than they actually do.

The family doctor conducts a special interview, one that looks like the most important in the life of the journalist where the journalist is totally focused on listening to what the interviewee says. Thus, the family doctor can not afford to ignore or forget the formal interview carried out in the hospital setting, there are times when you may need it, but in general, the family doctor will use a less formal interview, playing with the patient's confidence and being the most sophisticated of its own medical prescriptions.

The family doctor as a journalist should remember to adopt a comprehensive approach to the patient, and many problems are not only in the medical field and are not confined to a particular specialty. Sometimes the family doctor can become so concerned about the diagnostics that he forgets his communication skills.

The most common mistake in “making history” is to turn the interview into a “police interrogation” in which only partial information is collected and which is generally biased in terms of the patient's situation.

The “history” (recall) is not merely descriptive, but is an interpretive activity: the patient gives his version of the symptoms. The mere questioning transforms the patient into a passive observer, so that the results of the consultations may result in a worse situation: patient dissatisfaction, lack of compliance, and future unnecessary queries.

The family doctor and the journalist focus on “active listening,” which is partly a skill, partly an attitude of mind, and partly a personal attribute: it requires a concentration on the expression and manifestation of the patient.

## References

Balint JA. Brief Encounters: Speaking with Patients. *Ann Intern Med.*1999; 131: 231-234. http://www.annals.org/cgi/reprint/131/3/231.pdf.

Balint M, Hunt J, Joyce D, Marinker M, Woodcock J. Treatment or diagnosis. A study of repeat prescriptions in general practice. London: Tavistock Publications; 1984.

Gordon J. One to one teaching and feedback. *BMJ* 2003;326:543. http://www.bmj.com/content/326/7388/543.full?etoc=.

Gude T, Vaglum P, Anvik T, Baerheim A, Eide H, Fasmer OB, et al. Observed Communication Skills: How Do They Relate To The Consultation Content? A nation-wide study of graduate medical students seeing a standardized patient for a first-time consultation in a general practice setting. *BMC Medical Education* 2007, 7:43doi:10.1186/1472-6920-7-43. http://bmcmededuc.biomedcentral.com/articles/10.1186/1472-6920-7-43.

Maguire R. Active listening. *Student BMJ.* http://bmj.com/cgi/content/full/322/7302/S3-7302.

Rakel RE. Compassion and the art of family medicine: from Osler to Opran. JABFP 2000;13(6):440-448. http://www.medscape.com/viewarticle/405817.

*Chapter 46*

# The Family Doctor as a Naturalist

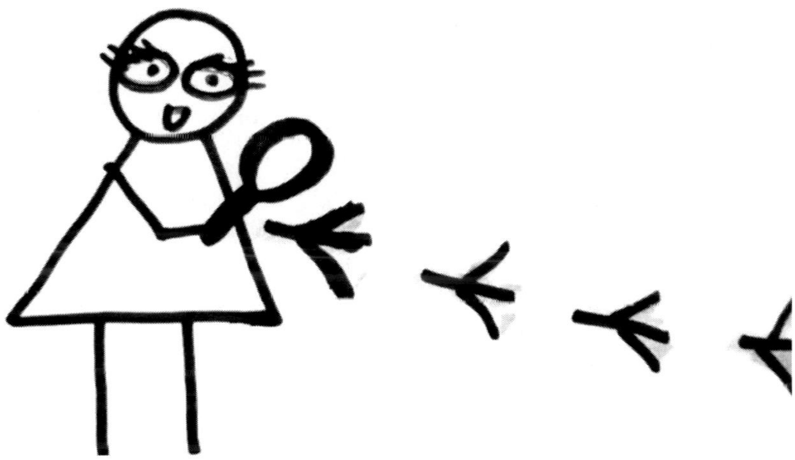

The naturalist carries a "field notebook" (his "history"). This is the main tool of every naturalist where he recorded his discoveries and impressions. Without it he would be likely to return home and fail to remember even half of what he had seen. The naturalist should always note the date, the place, the time and the weather. There may also be other useful data, for example, if it has been raining steadily several weeks, whether the autumn frost have begun, if the field is suffering a drought, or any other thing that he deems to be important or out of the ordinary and that could determine the behavior or appearance of some of the creatures. In addition, the naturalist looks for footprints and tracks.

The diagnostic process in family medicine can be understood as a means "to find a track, footprints, some traces." Every day, in the consultation, the diagnostic work of the family doctor is like that of the naturalist: he produces a record of the activities of the animal world that is printed in the landscape of the field, in the sand dunes of the beach and the desert, in the mud of the current in the river mouth, or after a snowfall. This is a printed record for anyone who wants to follow it; it is a vast map with clues and traces of immense variety and often wonderful clarity; it is an endless source of fascination for those who have eyes to see.

The diagnostic process of the family doctor is a mental operation through which the pathology is identified and the disease is evaluated. One of the great challenges faced by the family doctor is to assess the significance of certain symptoms and to diagnose. When the patient raises the problem, the family physician is faced with a plethora of data: the observations of the doctor himself, his prior knowledge of the patient, the contributions of the family, of other doctors, etc. There is so much information that cannot be analyzed all. Furthermore, different aspects of the information do not carry the same value. So, the family doctor responds to any information that has special meaning for him.

We can call evidence or "footprints" or "traces" to that kind of initial information. This evidence can be in the form of scars, signs, it may relate to a patient's behavior, age, previous history, context or ethnicity, companions, or requests for medical assistance.

In addition to identifying the tracks, the family doctor weighs their particular meaning. Within these traces or fingerprints, the track of "this fact should not be there" is especially useful in helping to identify the patient's problem or, too frequently, in ruling out other possible initial diagnoses, considering that often the family doctor must diagnose which problems they are not, rather than what they are.

How does the family doctor identify health problems/diseases for the traces, tracks, and footprints? The first problem is to decide if any trail has been left. The variety may seem puzzling and, as for the naturalist, "the wind or sun or rain may have ruined everything except the most recent footprints" — the previous treatment, the individual patient experience, the actions or strategies to relieve the patient's symptoms, variations in time, the appearance of new symptoms that can mask the early symptoms, etc.

After establishing the traces, the next problem is to discover when and why they appeared. Traces can provide information about what happened that cannot be obtained otherwise. More particularly, "the art of good tracker is to find something that is out of place." It's like what happened to Robinson Crusoe: how could that human footprint appear on a deserted island? It was a mystery.

From a particular trace or trail, an experienced family doctor will consider one or more hypothesis, as does the naturalist when he encounters a footprint in the sand — he can immediately, intuitively or automatically, see the direction of travel of the animal, if it is alone or accompanied, if it travels with a calf or with the whole family, if they were defending themselves against an enemy or fleeing and changing direction, if a large bird soared over the sand, or a predatory animal dragged his prey, or the versatility of the cranes in the sand on the beach, the sudden braking of the foxes, etc.

In other words, the family doctor works in the same way as the naturalist.

# References

Ennion EAR, Tinbergen N. Tracks. London: Oxford at the Clarendon Press; 1969.

http://apps.elsevier.es/watermark/ctl_servlet?_f=10&pident_articulo=90443461&pident_usuario=0&pcontactid=&pident_revista=27&ty=22&accion=L&origen=zonadelectura&web=www.elsevier.es&lan=es&fichero=27v47n09a90443461pdf001.pdf.

Marsé J. Rabos de lagartija. Barcelona: Planeta DeAgostini; 2002.

Turabián JL, Samarín-Ocampo E, Minier L, Pérez-Franco B. Learning concepts of diagnosis in family medicine: the ''mark Robinson sign'' – the traces that should not be there. Aten

Primaria. 2015; 47(9): 596-602. http://www.elsevier.es/ct-revista-atencion-primaria-27-articulo-aprendiendo-conceptos-del-diagnostico-medicina-90443461.

Turabian JL. Cuadernos de Medicina de Familia y Comunitaria. Una introducción a los principios de Medicina de Familia. Madrid: Díaz de Santos. 1995.

Chapter 47

# The Family Doctor as an Athlete Doing Rafting

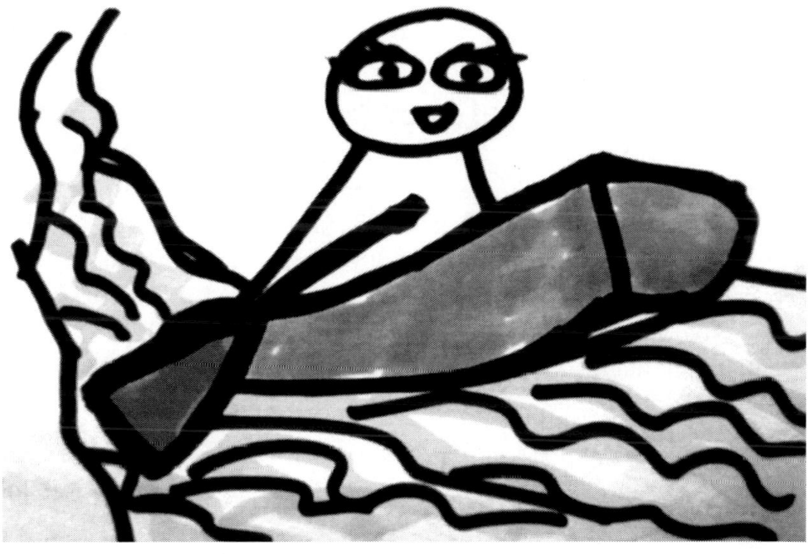

What is rafting? Rafting is one of the so-called risk sports, which is basically the rapid descent of rivers with a rowing boat. It entails coping with rapid water flow turning with the flow down the river. The feeling experienced during a rafting adventure is what makes it more appealing. Rafting requires no special physical condition other than the indispensable ability to swim.

The family doctor is like an athlete who goes rafting every day. The family doctor is rafting with speed along the "white-water consultations." The family doctor has to complete the consultation in 10 or maybe 15 minutes. There are perhaps 30 or 40 patients waiting. The river that leads us is the care maelstrom ... its waters are cold and murky and there are hidden rocks in the background in the form of problems, difficulties, anxieties, doubts, errors, conflicts, and so on.

The family doctor as an athlete rafting must be equipped for the "sport" and must know perfectly that stretch of the river because he has been there before. You will often see a problem that is difficult to overcome, and the boat hits a rock — it could tip if the occupant does not know how to control it. The family doctor knows that when hitting a rock he should not move his body backwards as this will make the boat capsize; on the contrary, he should place his weight forward and "face" the problem.

Rafting is difficult, but it can only be learned through practice, letting the river take you, whilst at the same time controlling the boat.

The athlete rafting and the family physician need time to reflect on how they are doing. In quiet moments, they can enjoy incredible landscapes and a sense (that is foreign to most) of knowing a river from within, getting carried away by the water and moving to the rhythm he imposes. But between trips there is not much time to think, to feel satisfied, or to grieve, as another patient enters the office and everything starts again.

Sometimes the river of family doctor's office brings little water, but when the rains are sufficiently abundant enough — epidemics of respiratory disease or the flu, the temporary peaks of gastroenteritis in the summer, cycles of anxiety and depression in times of economic recession — provide the required flow, and we can raft through the day at full speed!

The truth is that the sense of adventure to descend the rapids of the family medicine consultation is unique. But, of course, we need to know how to swim.

## References

Saura Llamas J. Formar médicos de familia: ¿Un rafting docente? *JANO* 1999; 57 (1304): 34.

Saura Llamas J. Mi experiencia docente en medicina familiar: Algunas habilidades para sobrevivir 22 años como Tutor. 10 Coloquio Internacional de Profesores Investigadores en Medicina Familiar. 30 marzo. 2012. http://www.investigacionenmedicina.org/conf_tutoria_2012/Mesa2_Espana.pdf.

WL Miller, Routine, ceremony, or drama: an exploratory study of the primary care clinical encounter, *J Fam Pract.* 1992; 34(3):289-96. http://www.ncbi.nlm.nih.gov/pubmed/1541955.

Chapter 48

# The Family Doctor as a Meteorologist

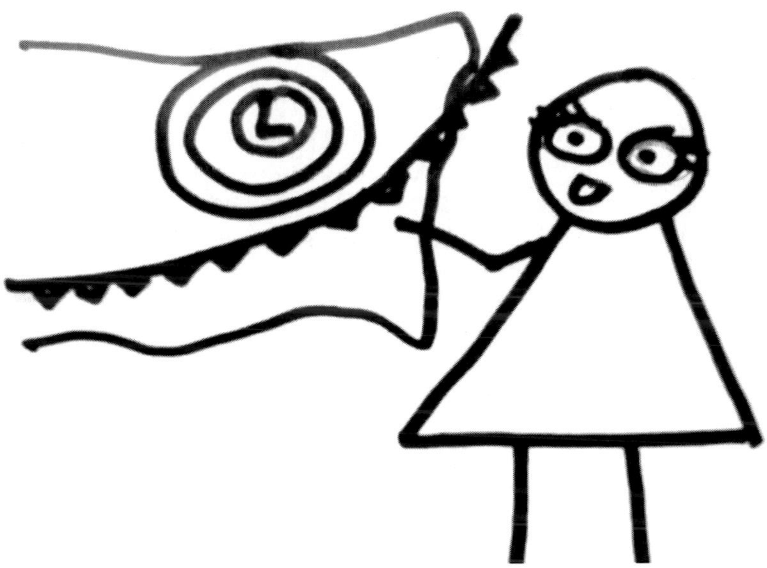

Meteorology is the science that studies the state of the atmosphere and meteors, i.e., atmospheric phenomena, particularly those related to the accuracy of the weather The science includes the study of daily variations in atmospheric conditions (which the family doctor might call "consultation by the current problem"), average and extreme conditions for long periods of time ("continuity of care and experience" for the GP), and the variation of meteorological elements in a small area (which the family doctor might refer to as "knowledge of small units — the family and its local community").

By studying the phenomena occurring in the atmosphere, meteorology is able to describe the climate, predict the weather, understand the interaction between the atmosphere and other subsystems, and so on. Knowledge of the weather and a future forecast of the same can help in critical situations.

All these concepts, the family doctor might call "contextualization," "relations," "stakeholders," and "prognosis." Medicine and meteorology also share their degrees of error but although there is generally a high degree of public understanding of the failures of meteorology, medical errors are not accepted and are commonly referred to as "malpractice."

Defining areas of weather risk as accurately as possible allows people to make alternative decisions in many sectors of socio-economic activity, such as the timely diversion of aircraft, ships and trucks, or planning activities in the open. In family medicine it is also possible to take aversive action, for example, identifying epidemiological risk groups allows for interventions in primary, secondary and tertiary prevention.

# References

El doctor Carlos J. Finlay Barrés y la meteorología. IV Congreso Nacional de Historia de la Ciencia y la Tecnología. La Habana, febrero de 2004. Cuadernos de Historia de la Salud Pública. http://bvs.sld.cu/revistas/his/his_99/his1099.htm.

Fry J. Common Diseases: Their Nature Incidence and Care.. Lancaster, England: MTP Press Limited; 1992.

http://www.amazon.co.uk/Cuadernos-medicina-familia-y-comunitaria/dp/8479781920.

Miguel García F. Factores de riesgo: una nada inocente ambigüedad en el corazón de la medicina actual. *Aten Primaria* 1998; 22(9):585-595.

Ricardo Batista Moliner. El médico de la familia en la vigilancia de salud. Rev Cubana Med Gen Integr 1997;13(1):59-62. http://www.bvs.sld.cu/revistas/mgi/vol13_1_97/mgi10197.htm.

Turabian JL. Cuadernos de Medicina de Familia y Comunitaria. Una introducción a los principios de Medicina de Familia. Madrid: Díaz de Santos. 1995.

*Chapter 49*

# The Family Doctor as an Educator

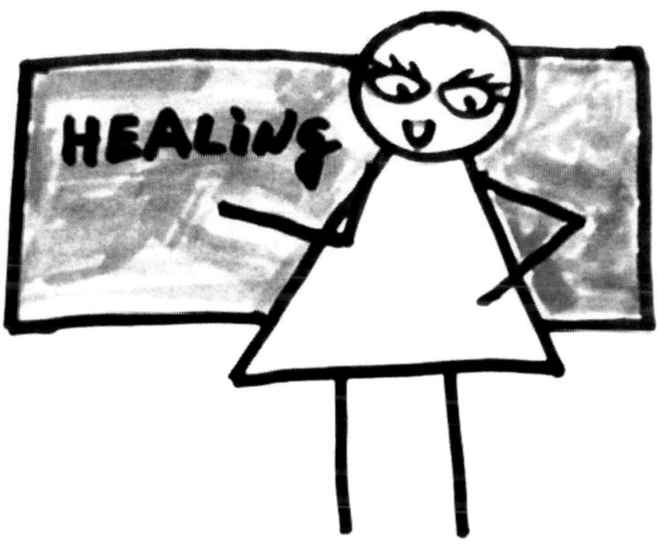


The term educator includes any person who takes action to educate, which is so closely linked to teachers in schools and universities. There are two types of teachers: first level, parents or tutors, teachers and schools; and a second level, friends, people from public life, the media, the Internet, etc. What about the family doctor? Does it make sense to talk about education in the context of the family doctor's office?

Imagine you are sick, so sick that you have to change your diet, your lifestyle and personal habits, and the doctor has prescribed, as a specific physical therapy, exercises and a number of drugs that you have to self-administer according to very detailed instructions. Now imagine trying to do all these things without being instructed on how to do them. This scenario presents an accurate idea of how important it is to understand the family doctor as a patient educator.

Addressing a large number of the problems in family medicine consultation is like conducting educational interventions to make the patient well again, as well as working on the context and actions that involve changing knowledge, attitudes, and the behaviors of patients. So, the family doctor should be seen as an educator. The clinical act is justified only insofar as it is also an educational act.

In a broad sense, education is considered as any combination of influences that change knowledge, attitudes, or behaviors. But the family doctor can apply three different educational tools:

1. A tool or informative model: this is about achieving knowledge (educational content of the "curriculum of the patient," which he must adapt). Its indicator is the knowledge of health/disease. The health outcomes are reducing morbidity and mortality and these are achieved through the doctor's methods, lectures, classes, informative tips, etc. Although health professionals usually attach great importance to the activities of imparting information to patients on consultation, studies indicate that their usefulness is limited.
2. A persuasive tool: information about motivation. Many educational theories are of this type and are derive from psychology (Health Belief Model, Reasoned Theory of Fishbein, Social Learning Theory, Theory of Locus of control, States of Change of Prochaska and DiClemente, etc.). The goals are to achieve behaviors that result in the avoidance of disease, as indicated by reducing smoking, increasing exercise, etc. The result is a reduction in morbidity and mortality. The method is persuasive medical advice.
3. A tool to promote empowerment: information that motivates and empowers, starting from the patient's needs. This model involves the educator building meanings and integrating or assimilating new material into the schemes of understanding that the patient already has. That is, what makes the content more or less significant is precisely the degree of insertion into previous schemes. It is "taking ideas instead of placing them." Thus, patients are helped to define their problems and to seek solutions themselves. The goal is increased individual control over health. The indicators of success are increased decision making, coping with problems, assertiveness, self-responsibility, cooperation, creativity, etc. The results are increased psycho-social status, development, empowerment, and positive health. The method is discussion, dialogue, group-work, games, simulations, group problem solving, case studies, community development, etc.

These three models are tools that allow us to provide treatment to the patient from different frames of reference. Finally, a balanced approach should prevail and there will be situations where it is preferable to perform a purely informative advice, in others, persuasion, and others seek empowerment, without forgetting that these models partly overlap.

Educators and practitioners should, in a pragmatic way, progress from simple to deeper insights.

## References

Bravo P, Edwards A, Barr PJ, Scholl I, Elwyn G, McAllister M, and the Cochrane Healthcare Quality Research Group, Cardiff University. Conceptualising patient empowerment: a mixed methods study. *BMC Health Serv Res.* 2015; 15:252. http://www.biomedcentral.com/1472-6963/15/252/abstract.

Turabian Fernandez JL. Are practitioners' teachers teaching the wrong things? The Spanish case. http://www.bmj.com/rapid-response/2011/10/28/are-practitioners-teachers-teaching-wrong-things-spanish-case.

Turabian JL, Perez Franco B. Consejos del médico de cabecera y estilos de vida saludables: □hay alternativa a la pasividad a la que nos obligan sus dificultades técnicas y éticas? *Med Clín* (Barc) 1998; 110:45.

Turabian JL, Pérez Franco B. Del consejo médico persuasivo al participativo en Medicina de Familia. Elementos para iniciar un debate. *MEDIFAM* 1995; 5(5):258-263.

Turabian JL, Perez Franco B. More Drugs to Cure Disorders in Human Relations? The Case of Addiction to Tobacco. Aten Primaria 2006;37(1):62-63. http://www.elsevier.es/es/revistas/atencion-primaria-27/mas-farmacos-curar-las-alteraciones-las-relaciones-13083930-cartas-al-director-2006.

Turabian JL, Perez Franco B. Too many theories of health promotion? *Med Clin* 2006; 126(5):198. http://www.elsevier.es/es/revistas/medicina-clinica-2/demasiadas-teorias-promocion-salud-13084544-cartas-al-editor-2006.

Turabian JL, Perez Franco B. Utilidad y límites de la edcuación sanitaria. *FMC* 1998; 5(7): 419-421.

Chapter 50

# The Family Doctor as the Painter Josef Albers

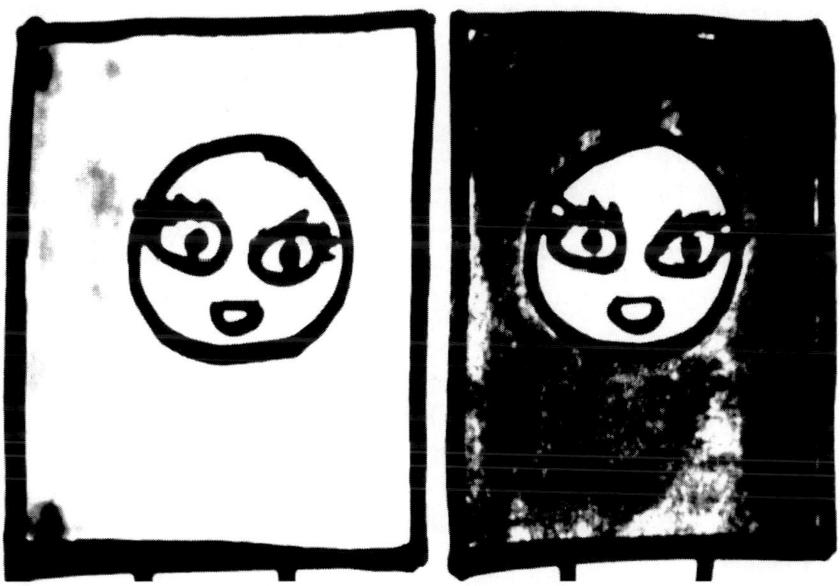

Albers developed an experimental way to study and teach about color. This was based on the idea that only by observing color in context can you begin to understand its nature. From here he could conclude that color is unstable, and susceptible to change depending on its proximity to other colors. Therefore, there is not a valid formula for color selection.

For the family doctor the diagnosis is made using a similar mechanism. The diagnosis is intended to highlight a picture on a background, "to recognize the contrast edges." Thus, the same problem takes different forms depending on the background — different diagnoses according to different contexts. Through to stand out a picture on a background ("contextualize").

For Albers, two green squares, one of them inside the other square white, and another inside square black one, both have the same green color, but the second seems darker.

A color can acquire two different faces. If we have two pink squares of exactly the same color (equal hue, brightness and value), one inside other square red, and another within a square blue, we perceive different shades of pink squares. This occurs because the pink color is contextually situated between the two background colors. The more different these background colors are from each other, the greater the influence on the color placed inside them. Likewise, two completely different colors may look like the same color when interacting with the colors alongside them.

In the world of Albers, free colors became orchestral sounds, cooking ingredients, tastes, geographic locations, and theater actors. The colors tell of other colors, some colors dominate others, some colors are dictatorships, and other colors are democracies. Some are jealous of others; others breathe together, some colors are happy, and even make love to each other. The related colors become nieces, nephews, second cousins, or children that reflect the qualities of their parents. Albers' color theory focused on the dynamic and changing nature of color in relation to its contexts: cloudy and vibrant colors when they are next to each other, and modified in tonal intensity and depth in three dimensional spaces.

For Albers, as well as the family doctor, it can be seen that same color (a health problem) causes completely different effects depending on the environment (personal, family, work, community, context). The family doctor has to put the symptom in context. The symptom "depends" on its environment.

Albers explained that "all backgrounds subtract (absorbs) the hue of the colors they contain, and therefore affect them. It follows that any diversity among colors, either in tone or in chiaroscuro relationship, can be visually reduced, if not eliminated, if these colors are placed on a background of equal quality. The family doctor should be aware of the "brightness of the background." The family doctor has to try to find those "colors" that are more susceptible to influence and distinguish them from those that are influenced.

## References

Albers J. La interacción del color. Madrid: Alianza Forma; 1979.

Friedler J, Feierabend P, Bauhaus, London: Ullman, 2010.

Go Now (film). Wikipedia. [homepage on the Internet]. https://en.wikipedia.org/wiki/Go_Now_(film).

Horowitz FA, Danilowitz B, Albers J: To Open Eyes: The Bauhaus, Black Mountain College, and Yale, London: Phaidon, 2006.

The Josef & Anni Albers Foundation. http://www.albersfoundation.org/.

Turabian JL, Perez Franco B. Atención médica individual con orientación comunitaria-Atención contextualizada: la figura es el fondo. Revista Clínica Electrónica en Atención Primaria. http://www.fbjoseplaporte.org/rceap/articulo2.php?idnum=16&art=08.

Wick R. La pedagogía de la Bauhaus, Barcelona: Alianza, 2000.

Wilson HJ. The myth of objectivity: is medicine moving towards a social constructivist medical paradigm? Fam Pract 2000;17:203-9. http://fampra.oxfordjournals.org/content/17/2/203.full.

*Chapter 51*

# The Family Doctor as a Fisherman Rather Than Hunter

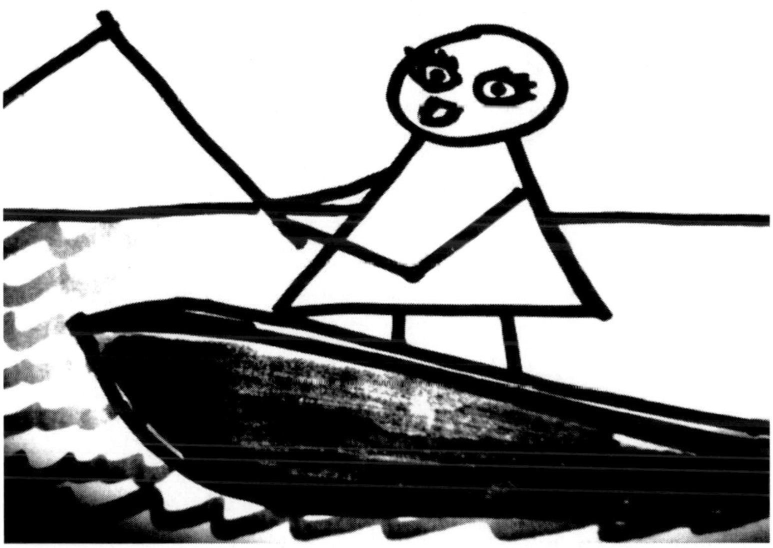

"One young man said at the end of the conference that gave the old professor:

I'd like to ask you a question that has been suggested to me by your important conference..."

"Whilst the old professor was listening to the question, a ray of light illuminated his papers. Yes, the question was transcendental, and the young man had captured the essence of what was a really important question. For the teacher, that question was as like a curtain being drawn aside. The person who opens the curtain could be dazzled by what appeared behind it, but the teacher was now perfectly clear. The teacher had spent a great deal of times without noticing that hole in his theories. It was like being lost in a maze and suddenly seeing the way out. The teacher suddenly saw everything perfectly clearly."

Questions have always been the classic means of obtaining information from others. We can use them to obtain information about ourselves or to direct our search. This is the basis of the "Socratic method." A question is an instrument to draw attention.

There are two types of questions:

1. Fishing questions
2. Hunting questions.

When we go fishing we put the bait into the water and do not know what we will get. A fishing question can have many answers. It is an open question: "What, how ...?" Asking open-ended questions and using open sentences is like saying, "continue." The family doctor has to ask open or "fishing" questions to identify the patient's needs, and he listen carefully to the patient's answers to help him understand the problem as experienced by the affected person. The family doctor has to be aware of what "fishing with cane."

When we go hunting we aiming at something in particular. We do not throw our weapons into the air waiting for a bird to pass our way. Hunting questions have a known target; they are confirmation questions. We have an idea about something and we want to check it. They are closed questions that are answered with "yes" or "no."

Asking questions uses a combination of fishing and hunting techniques. It is also necessary that we set aside the time to catch something: fish do not always bite immediately we put the bait in the water. The family doctor needs patience to listen constructively. We often miss important information because we pass too quickly onto the next question. If the family doctor asks a lot of questions, he spends time thinking about the next question instead of thinking about the answers.

The family doctor, especially at the beginning of the interview, has do ask open-ended questions — those that ask what, when, who, why, where and how. The family doctor has to be a fisherman, putting the bait into the water and being attentive, not knowing what is going to bite. Moreover, these questions may also to illuminate to doctor for the clarification of the diagnostic process. "Questions fishing" are made by the family doctor to the patient, and also himself.

Some questions that can guide medical research in understanding the whole person are: at what point in the family life cycle is the patient? (e.g., starting a family, retirement), where is each family member in their life cycle? (teen, middle age), how does the disease affects the achievement of the different tasks of the family, what kinds of diseases have the family experienced, what kind of support has been mobilized in the past to cope with family disease, has a support network now been established?

## References

De Bono E. Aprende a pensar por ti mismo. Barcelona: Paidós; 1977.

https://uthscsa.influuent.utsystem.edu/en/publications/have-you-really-addressed-your-patients-concerns(beef46ce-2210-41cb-b1ba-d0ab7fa474c8).html.

JANO 2004; LXVI (1515): 10. http://www.jano.es/ficheros/sumarios/1/66/1515/10/1v66n1515a13060124pdf001.pdf.

Ronald M. Epstein RN, Mauksch L, Carroll J, Jaén CR. Have You Really Addressed Your Patient's Concerns? *Fam Pract Manag.* 2008;15(3):35-40.

Sampedro JL. Congreso en Estocolmo. Barcelona: Plaza y Janés Editores, S.A.; 1997.

Saxton H. Asking the right questions. BMJ 2001;323:1393. http://www.bmj.com/content/323/7326/1393.full/.

Turabian JL. La ley del embudo inverso y los éxitos que son fracasos/.

Chapter 52

# The Family Doctor as a Pre-Raphaelite Painter

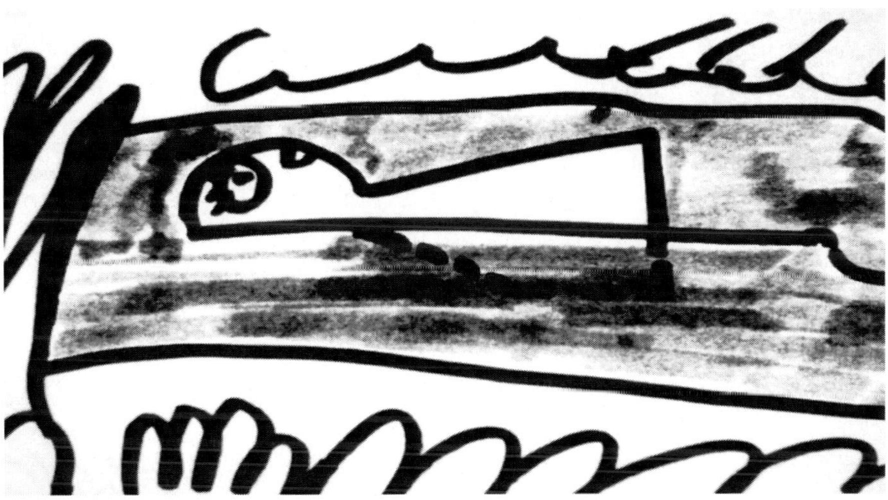

The family physician must go from external to internal values, from sociology to psychology. He should look inwardly abroad or convert the outside to the inside.

Some painters like Rossetti, Burne Jones, and the Pre-Raphaelite followers, Bocklin, Stuck and his successors, were seekers of the inside on the outside and they were placed in the realm of myth and legend, like the symbolist painter Segantini, who worked natural forms in the smallest detail (e.g., ridges, rocks, animals, etc.).

According to Cézanne (the researcher of the new law of pictorial form), the problem was raised by another road, closer to the pure pictorial means. He transformed a teacup into a living being, or better still, he acknowledged that the cup was a living being. Cézanne had the idea of reaching into the deep sense of things through their individual temperament.

The external appearance (shape, sociological) is an expression of inner content (psychic, spiritual, soul). The inevitable relationship between color and form leads us to observe the effects of form over color. The form itself, even when it is completely abstract and looks like a geometric shape, has its own internal sound; it is a spiritual entity. A triangle, for example, is one of those entities with its own spiritual perfume. When this form is related to other forms, this perfume is differentiated and acquires nuances. A yellow triangle and a green triangle are completely different entities and act quite differently. It is a subjective substance in an objective housing. Every form has an internal content. The external form, is therefore the expression of the inner content.

For example, Rossetti painted the Annunciation in such a way that the atmosphere, the attitude of the characters, and the compositional form, obtained a pictorial result that is closer to the mystery of symbols that the own mystery of the painted scene. In this way, the virginal purity is reflected in the white walls, the curtains, the lilies, and the clothes of Mary and the angel.

The family doctor has to remember that personal characteristics create contexts. The consequences of disability, ethnicity, sex, gender, age, temperament, behavior, and attitudes create contexts within which the patient moves. The patient's health problem is reflected in his atmosphere. These external values that we see at first glance should lead us to the inner values of the patient. Individual characteristics modify, produce, or are reflected in its context. The person chooses a particular context that is paired with their personal characteristics.

Furthermore, the Pre-Raphaelite painters worked each frame by areas, in a very delicate way, in order to capture even the smallest detail. Similarly, the family doctor has to treat the patient by trying to capture the smallest details, and this may require using "work areas," perhaps from the sociological to the psychological, seeking the visible representation of sensations.

## References

Bowes JM, Hayes A. Children, familias, and communities. Contexts and consequences. Victoria, Australia: Oxford University Press; 1999.

De lo espiritual en el arte. Barcelona: Barral Editores, S. A.; 1982.

http://zl.elsevier.es/es/revista/semergen-medicina-familia-40/resumen/viaje-lo-esencial-invisible-aspectos-90279179.

Turabian JL, Perez Franco B. Journey to what is essentially invisible: Pysochosocial aspects of disease. Semergen. 2014;40:65-72.

Waters W. Edward Burne-Jones. Oxford: Shire Publications Ltd; 1973.

Chapter 53

# The Family Doctor as the Genie in Aladdin's Lamp

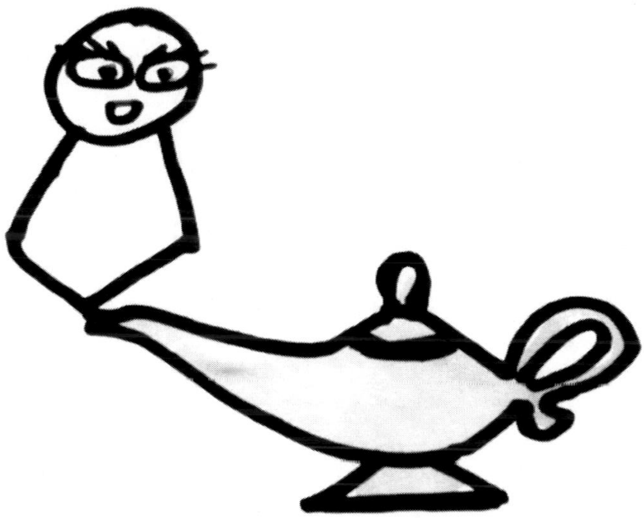

Aladdin is one of the Syrian origin stories of the *Thousand and One Nights* (although its characters are from the Far East). Aladdin, who has the lamp, discovers that he can summon a genie that is required to serve the person holding the "magic lamp."

It is true that the social demand in our context is biological. The economic interests of the pharmaceutical industry and technology impact on government budgets and manipulate politicians, health experts, research results, scientific societies, study plans, media and citizens, etc. The family doctor may be more effectual when he does his work with pleasure, achieving emotional gratification at the micro level of the consultation where he treats people and their emotions and pathologies in contexts.

Each family doctor attends to approximately 2,000 patients. Depending on how the family physician is professionally related to the patients, they come to perceive what we call the bio-psychosocial individual and despite the social and hospital influence, patients ask their family doctor, for example, whether they have to take the drugs prescribed by the specialist, or whether they have to accept surgery..., and in the end they do what their family doctor tells them! That is, patients often rely more on their family doctor than they do on the super specialist.

The construction of doctor-patient trust and the bio-psychosocial approach carried out in the office of the family doctor is like a small Aladdin's lamp — in the relationship with the patient we rub the human, the emotional, the bio-psychosocial, the integrated ... and a genie emerges that grants our desires!

Every patient is a citizen (and voter) and each family doctor has 2,000 people in his care, and, furthermore, each of these patients is immersed in their family and community relationships. So the effect of Aladdin's lamp can multiply without realizing it!

The family doctor is not pessimistic and if he finally has to accept that state of mind, he is an "active pessimist."

Family physicians are the "genies of the lamp." We just have to rub the lamp.

## References

Cebrià Andreu J. Emociones y motivaciones en las consultas médicas (II). Jano 2001;LX:2119-20.

De Bono E. Opportunities. Middlesex: Penguin Books; 1981.

http://zl.elsevier.es/es/revista/atencion-primaria-27/la-emocion-intuicion-como-herramientas-gestionar-incertidumbre-13073417-special-article-2005.

Turabián Fernández JL, Pérez Franco B. Notes on "resolutivity" and "cure" in family medicine. Aten Primaria. 2003; 32:296-9. http://www.elsevier.es/es-revista-atencion-primaria-27-articulo-apuntes-resolutividad-cura-medicina-familia-13051598.

Turabian JL, Perez Franco B. Emotion and Intuition as Tools to Deal With Uncertainty When Taking Decisions in Family Practice. *Aten Primaria* 2005;35(6):306-310.

*Chapter 54*

# The Family Doctor as a Sea Turtle

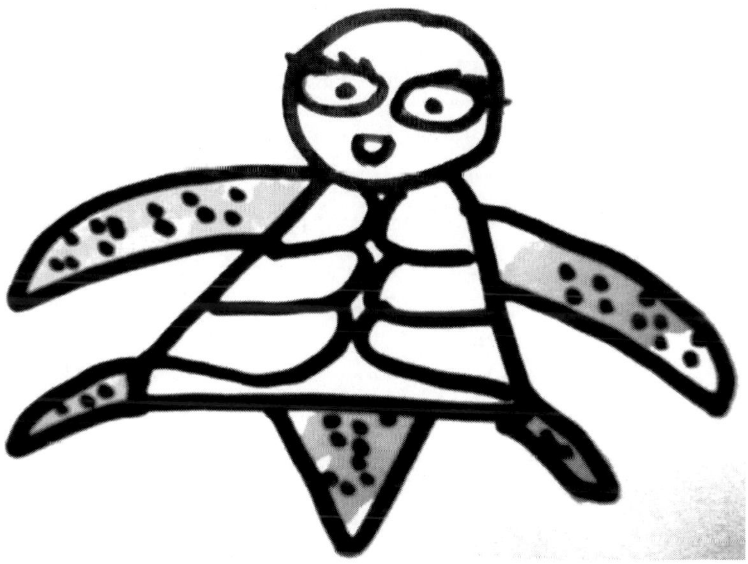

Sea turtles are able to perform very long trips on the open sea and to reach their destination with incredible precision. What do turtles use to navigate in the amplitude of the oceans? It is still a mystery today as to how they find their way to such small and remote locations in the ocean with no apparent reference points. Sea turtles can travel thousands of kilometers across the ocean — from the Ascension Islands to the coast of Brazil — and they seem to follow the same routes; some are diverted along the way but are able to adjust their direction to reach their destination. Of course, they do not navigate by viewing the coastline; they travel towards their destination for several hundred kilometers before seeing the coast.

The turtles swim at an average speed of 2 to 3 kilometers per hour, equivalent to a stroll leisurely pace, or in the sea, to a travel in a rowboat. Sea turtles swim both day and night, in daylight or after dark, under a starlit open sky or in the absence of sun, stars and moon. So, unlike many other migratory creatures, such as birds and monarch butterflies, for example, who are guided by the sun or the stars, sea turtles can manage without these elements. The mechanisms that allow the turtles to keep to the route in the ocean remain a mystery.

Family physicians are able to understand the full impact of the disease (neurological, cardiac, etc.), and determine the diagnosis, treatment, prognosis, clinical course, and severity in a particular individual, without having “protocols” for each health problem in each patient. What do family physicians use to navigate in the amplitude of the clinic? How in the middle of the clinic do they find, without apparent reference points, such concrete and small data?

When we see illness out its psychosocial context, it is as to have “a fish out of water.” When the family physician diagnoses, treats, and assesses the prognosis of a health problem, even a seemingly biomedical pathology, regardless of the psychosocial global context, it is like “a fish out of water.” All diseases are like pebbles polished by the river, which can be of enormous dimensions and different shapes, but in some way they are all the same due to the effect of context: the variable, which produces the distinctive element is the context — the force of the river, its flow, its meanders, its slopes. Actually, biomedical pathologies that may appear to be very different — heart failure, asthma, breast cancer, etc. — are the same. They are only different in their diagnosis, prognosis and course of treatment because of their context.

Family physicians use their knowledge of the psychosocial context of the patient as a mechanism to guide the uncertainty of the diagnosis, clinical course, treatment, and prognosis of disease.

## References

Ghione S. La isla de las tortugas. Viaje a Ascensión. Barcelona: Ediciones Península; 2002.

Kerns RD, Curley AL. A biopsychosocial approach to illness and family: neurological diseases across the life span. En: Turk DC, Kerns RD (Editores). Health, illness, and families. A life-span perspective. New York: John Wiley and Sons; 1985.

Turabian Fernandez JL, Perez Franco B. Do family doctors seem like turtles? Semergen. 2008;34(8):373-374. http://www.elsevier.es/es/revistas/semergen-medicina-general--familia-40/se-parecen-los-medicos-familia-las-tortugas-13127213-editoriales-2008.

*Chapter 55*

# The Family Doctor as a Sculptor

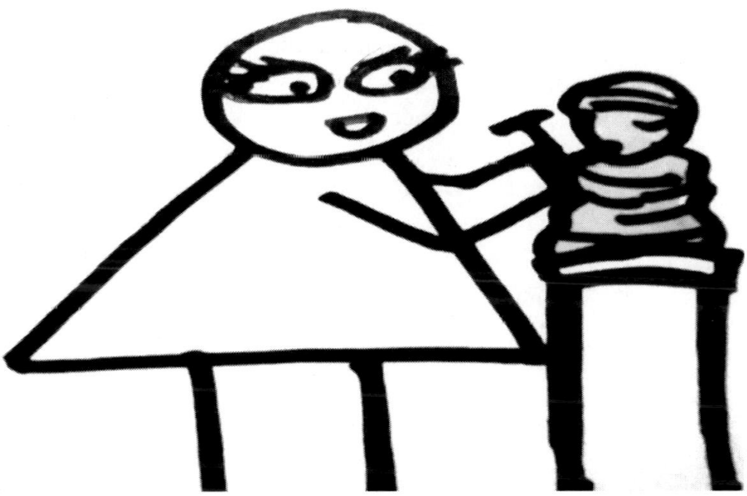

The family doctor does not "do" diagnostics: he is building and re-building diagnostics. The diagnosis is not presented as a final package. Rather, it is built and re-built like carving a sculpture. The diagnostic process is imprecise and continually evolving. The diagnosis must always be in motion, it is dynamic, open, and never stabilizes (chaotic context); there is no end point.

As a sculptor, the family doctor faces the future statue is currently only a rough stone block, without modelling clay, wood, or other materials. Very different patients consult the family physician: they are different —iron, bronze, sandstone materials, lead, wax, plaster, clay, resin, plastic, fibreglass, concrete, limestone, marble, alabaster, granite, quartz, jade, stucco, gold, silver, steel, wood, ivory, concrete — and the family doctor will have to use appropriate methods to sculpt these material differences!

The craftsman has to produce a sculpture, removing anything that hides the beauty of the statue. The family doctor uses a process of taking a medical history and diagnostic through which he has to polish the original stone and release its beauty. To do this, the doctor has to accept changes, movements, and continuous evolution, and he will try to understand the main or essential data. The sculptor, like the medical history and diagnosis, will model, sculpting, draining, chiselling, embossing, stamping, welding, or stuffing gradually his work.

Sculpture and medical history, is molded, is removed, is filled ... until it is "ends" at an arbitrary point, from which can restart the process ... But meanwhile, the visit ends and the history or diagnosis, like the sculpture, is placed in the gallery on paper or in a electronic file, waiting to be reconstructed when the patient returns.

The sculptor and the family doctor cannot modified stone or other materials and achieve a masterpiece if they have not first changed their way of thinking. Both have to try to understand the essentials. The sculptor, like the family doctor, removes everything that is superfluous and reduces the material to its purest form.

## References

Bulgákov M. Morfina. Barcelona: Anagrama; 2002.

http://myslide.es/documents/hacp-electronica-sopa-con-tenedor-cuad-gestion-2004.html.

http://www.amazon.co.uk/Cuadernos-medicina-familia-y-comunitaria/dp/8479781920.

Norman G, Barraclough K, Dolovich L, Price D. Iterative diagnosis. BMJ. 2009;339:b3490. http://www.bmj.com/content/339/bmj.b3490?etoc=.

Turabian fernández JL, Pérez Franco B. La historia clínica electrónica: ¿comer sopa con tenedor? Cuadernos de Gestión 2004;10(4):175-188.

Turabian JL. Cuadernos de Medicina de Familia y Comunitaria. Una introducción a los principios de Medicina de Familia. Madrid: Díaz de Santos. 1995.

*Chapter 56*

# The Family Doctor as a "Middle of the Road Beatnik"

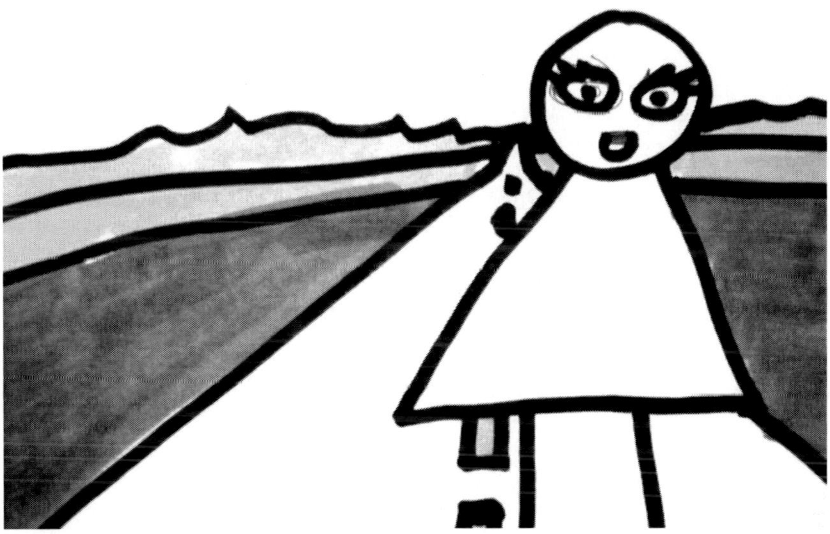

Jack Kerouac's semi-autobiographical novel, *On the Road* (1957), is one of the most popular and fundamental statements of the early Beat movement. It tells the story of a group of friends travelling across North America in search of new and intense experiences. It is a novel that has many similarities with the work of the family doctor.

Family doctors in training soon learn that the general hospital is separated from the psychiatric hospital by a "road." On the left side of the road is the large general hospital complex that has grown even more over recent years. On the right side of the road are the remains of the psychiatric hospital. The mind and the emotions are on the right and the body and the mathematical sciences are to the left of the road. Patients continually make dualistic choices and the structure is ready to facilitate this separation. The family doctor is in the uncomfortable area in the middle, between biomedical medicine and psychiatry, between evidence-based medicine and emotions. Being in "middle of the road" is a very dangerous place, and it is normal to feel "threatened" here.

The family doctor sees many patients who will speak first of their bodies — they have asthenia, pain, weakness, abdominal disorders, etc. — and the doctor tends to see them on the left side of the road. Some will speak of sadness, fear, anger, frustration, anxiety, hopelessness, and these are seen on the right side of the road. But if the family doctor asks to these patients about their physical symptoms, the most admit having them. Moreover, if the family doctor asks the former type of patients about their emotional state, most of them admit stress and emotional problems.

Three decades of studies and research have shown us beyond any reasonable doubt that in symptoms of illness, the mind and body are inextricably interrelated: if you have "physical" symptoms you almost invariably have similar levels of "psychological" symptoms and vice versa. That both psychological and social factors contribute to disease is clear, and they are very much related to quality of life. Understanding both provides a level of excellence in the medical approach.

Yet medical practice remains dualistic, perhaps becoming more intense and more dualistic. The principle of first solving the "physical" and then addressing the psychosocial, remains the basis of modern medical practice. The biomedical approach to disease is hugely beneficial and its progress is accelerating with genetic and neurochemical knowledge. At the same time there is a great paradox. While we have never been so healthy and live to an increasingly older age, we seem to be more concerned about our health and suffer more chronic diseases than ever before. Family medicine is the academic discipline that unites this body-mind duality.

Family physicians need to learn to be "in the middle of the road."

## References

Balner H (Editor), DeVries MJ, Engel GL, Goodkin IK, LeShan L, Lynch JJ, Rosch PJ, Stikker A. A New Medical Model: A Challenge for Biomedicine? Publications of The Helen Dowling Institute for Biopsychosocial Medicine, 1. Amsterdam: Swets & Zeitlinger B.V. Amsterdam/Lisse; 1990.

Bracken P, Thomas P. Time to move beyond the mind-body split. BMJ 2002;325:1433. http://bmj.com/cgi/content/full/325/7378/1433?etoc.

Engel, 1980; St Claire Lindsay. Rival Truths. Common sense and social psychological explanations in health and illness. New York: Psichology Press. Taylor & Francis Group; 2003.

Kerouac J. On the Road. London: Penguin; 2000.

Turabian Fernandez JL En medio de la carretera. JANO 2008, 27 de junio.

White P (editor). Biopsychosocial medicine. An integrated approach to understanding illness. Oxford: Oxford Univesity Press; 2005.

*Chapter 57*

# The Family Doctor as a Reader of Patients

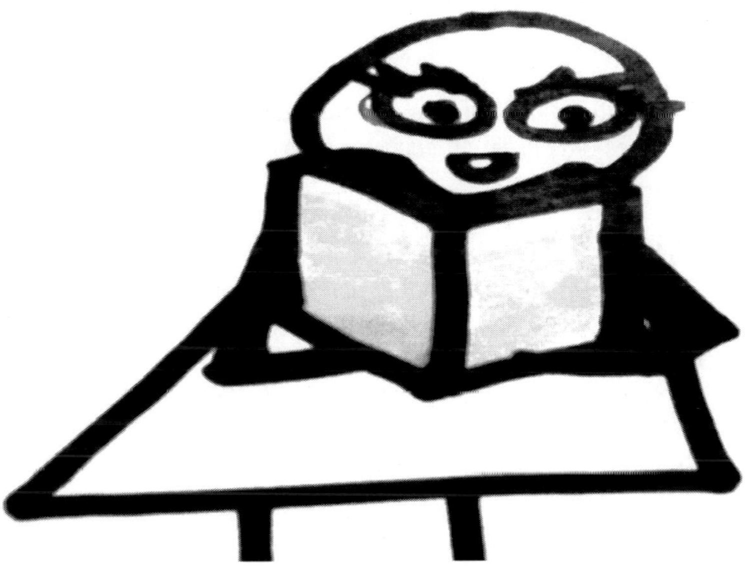

The patient is a text to be read. Patients are texts that are examined and studied by the clinician. Sometimes they can be read like a book, the text of a newspaper article, or a piece of prose that explains the issue directly. At other times, the stories of patients resemble novels or poems, written with more complicated words, the meaning of which are not always immediately understood. Doctors are readers of these texts.

The patient's history is a text produced by the disease. The patient and the doctor are co-authors of that text. The most common form of narrative or biography of the disease is the medical history; it is the official text of the experience of illness. The history occurs in collaboration (albeit explicit or implicit) and is therefore a product of both the physician and patient. There is a continuum of information for understanding the narrative of the disease, including clinical notes, interviews, transcripts of audio-tapes, diaries, video recordings, etc.

The novel, poetry, and theatre provide medicine with visions of human experience. The human mind is inevitably imperfect, but focusing medical attention on the patient's narrative allows us insights into their circumstances. As wise family physicians we need, first, to understand and then to imagine the stories that our patients tell, and to which, healthy or sick, they should return after consultation. The diagnosis is encoded in the narrative — in the story told by the patient. In addition, understanding the story told by the patient has profound therapeutic implications.

In respect of patients, doctors have learned the importance of narrative — the story. More and more doctors write about their consultations with non-medical scientists, but they do this in narrative terms thus highlighting human interactions — the personal and emotional aspects of the care given to individual patients — and that helps them to understand the lives of patients.

Family physicians can "read" patients as they might read a "biography": the patient can be read in terms of the past, which takes into account details such as marital stress, job loss, illness of a child, and so on. For example, elevated blood pressure can be recorded prior to experiencing difficult circumstances. The patient can be read as a "verse" with a rhyme that is continually repeated and which we expect to appear in the next verse. Is the patient a sonnet? There are aspects of the patient's biography that are repeated; a pattern that repeats itself (as in rhymes).

Is it possible for the patient to be read as a "short story"? The patient makes many visits but in each of them focuses on a different concern; such once patient is a frequent consultant with many short visits for various topics.

Is it possible for the patient to be read as a "sentimental novel"? The story focuses on the relationship and the end of the story must be positive, embracing nature, love, ingenuity, passion and melancholy. Or perhaps the reading may be that entailed in a "cowboy novel set in the American West" where the antagonism between the characters is resolved by a duel with pistols and machetes.

Alternatively, the patient may be a "Byzantine novel" characterized by the accumulation of improbable adventures and episodes. Or the patient may be a "Gothic novel" with ruins, churches, monasteries, mystery and intrigue. Or he is a "detective novel" whose topic is the resolution of an enigma. Or he is a "psychological novel" that describes psychological conflicts. Or the patient is a novel of "science fiction" with stories that show the impact of scientific and technological advances. Or a "comedy" that is characterized by main characters who, when faced with the difficulties of everyday life are driven to happy endings by their own defects. Or a "drama or tragedy": a patient with terminal cancer. Or a "cartoon" with a series of drawings that constitute a story. Or the patient is a "travel book" with the experiences and observations of a traveller.

## References

Donnelly WJ. Patients' Stories as Narrative. JAMA. 2002;287(4):447-448. http://jama.jamanetwork.com/article.aspx?articleid=1031700.

Estroff SE. Whose story is it anyway? Autority, voice, and responsability in narratives of chronic illness. En: Chronic Ilness. From experience to policy. Edited by Tomms SK,

Barnard D, and Carson RA. Bloomington and Indianapolis: Indiana University Press; 1995.

Greenhalgh T, Hurwitz B. (Editors). Narrative Based Medicine. Dialogue and discouse in clinical practice. London: BMJ Books; 1998.

Hunter KM. Doctors' Stories. The narrative structure of medical knowledge. Princeton, New Jersey: Princeton University Press; 1991.

Sacks O. El hombre que confundió a su mujer con un sombrero." Barcelona: Muchnik; 1991.

Sacks O. The Island of Colour-blind. London: Picador; 1996.

Sampedro JL. Monte Sinaí. Barcelona: Plaza & Janés Editores, S.A.; 1998.

Saxton M, Howe F. With Wings. An anthology of literature by women with disabilities. London: Virago Press Limited; 1988.

Turabian Fernandez JL. La historia de cada paciente es un texto que se lee. JANO 2009.

*Chapter 58*

# The Family Doctor as a Magpie

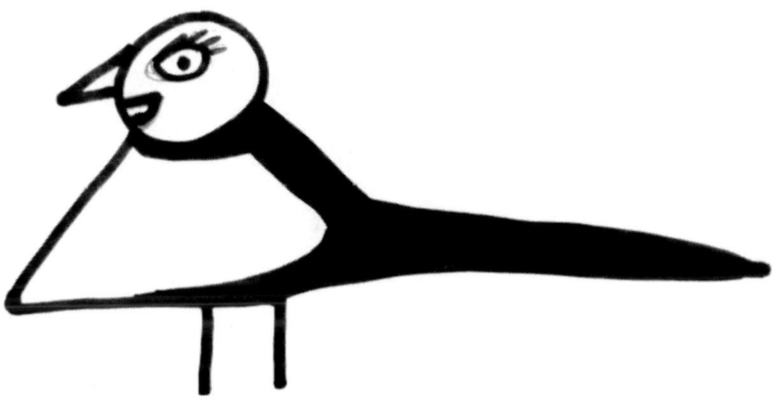

The family physician works as birds do when building their nests: thoroughly intertwining twigs and bits of straw, moss and other materials, and lining the inside with feathers, tufts of wool or grass or vegetables gathered from various places.

The family physician follows the system or style of magpies — threading, connecting objects, facts, historical periods, the results of physical examinations, of laboratory tests, hospital specialists' opinions — and arranges them in the sequence that seems most effective.

The patient goes to the doctors' office one day, his wife visits the office another day, or the children come, or the patient is accompanied by one of them. On each of these visits the family doctor takes a twig, a piece of straw, a bit of moss, or a flake of wool and gradually builds a knowledge of that person which will be very useful to subsequently make a correct diagnosis and prescribe appropriate treatment. It may take patience to build that knowledge, as it does for birds where their patience is notable and ingenuity and skill are displayed when building their nests. Family physicians are also tireless in developing a body of knowledge about their patients, and they continue to improve their skills with experience.

However, collection of such information should not be done in any way; should not be made inadequate or untimely questions. Like the bird, the family doctor does not build a "nest" in any old way, or anywhere, but seeks the right method and selects the most appropriate materials. These "nests" are the knowledge that the family doctor acquires about the patient over time; may seem weak, but on the contrary, is strong. All the knowledge of a patient can be "subjective" or "soft," and comes from various sources that have been intertwined by the family doctor; yet ultimately, this knowledge is stronger than the called "objective."

# References

Focault M. El nacimiento de la clínica. Una arqueología de la mirada médica. Mexico: Siglo XXI Editores; 1991.

Lázaro J. Medicina científica y medicina personal. JANO. 2002; 63 (1447): 94-95.

Morris J. Venecia. Barcelona: Ediciones Península; 2002.

Panofsky E. La perspectiva como forma simbólica. Barcelona: Tusquets Editor; 1978.

Vilar S. La nueva racionalidad. Comprender la complejidad con métodos transdisciplinarios. Barcelona: Editorial Kairos; 1997.

*Chapter 59*

# The Family Doctor as a Taoist Master

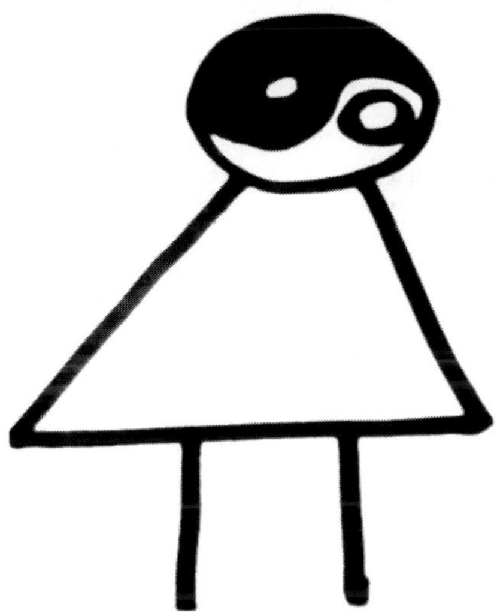

The Taoist theory of eternal immortality is about moving. It is the journey, not the arrival that is worthy of interest. The process is vital. The family doctor is also more interested in the process than the result.

As for the Taoist, the work of the family doctor is dedicated to the worship of the imperfect. Just as the lack of symmetry characterizes Japanese art objects, and greater importance is attached to how to seek perfection itself, the family doctor knows that his work will never be perfect and he seeks that perfection in the process of continued relationship with patients and their context. The true beauty only comes when mentally incompleteness is completed.

Thus, landscapes and flowers have become the favourites themes of the Taoist painting, rather than the human figure whose presence is only in the mind of the beholder. The family physician also looks first, and attaches great importance, to the landscape and flowers: the context of the patient.

Tao literally means path. But often it is attributed other meanings such as the Absolute Law, Nature, Supreme Reason, infinity, the fugitive, evanescent, and the Vanishing Return. The Tao is in the passage rather than the path.

Taoism, as family medicine, is the "art of being in the world" and the art of life is to be in the middle. According to Taoists, the secret to success in the drama of life lies in keeping things in proportion.

For the Taoists, as for family doctors, our role is the "worship of the imperfect." the vision of all is not to be drowned out by the individual selfishness. Lao Tse demonstrated that idea with his metaphor of emptiness: the context "will find, for example, the reality of a room, not on the roof and walls, but in the limited space of these entities. The jug is useful because it is a space that contains water and not because of the shape of the vessel or clay that the potter molded. The vacuum is powerful because it can enclose everything. Movement is only possible in a vacuum."

The Taoist accepts the world as it is, struggling to discover the beauty in this world of misery and boredom. The Sung allegory of the Three Vinegar Tasters admirably explains the trend of the three doctrines [Buddhism, Confucianism, Taoism]. One day, Buddha, Confucius, and Lao Tse were talking about a jar of vinegar (symbol of life), into which each one dipped a finger to taste the liquid. Confucius found it acid; Buddha found it bitter; and Lao Tse found it sweet.

The family physician is a jiu-jitsu fighter. Jujitsu, the art of self-defence, is named after a passage from the *Tao Te Ching*. In jiu-jitsu the fighter patiently strives to attract and absorb the force of the adversary using non-resistance, that is, using the vacuum, and reserving his own strength for the final attack, which is what decides the outcome. The principle of vacuum applied to art, reaches its predominant value in the suggestion. By not saying everything, the family doctor, like the Taoist artist, gives the patient or the viewer the chance to integrate the idea, and to thus captivate our attention to the point where we become part of the masterpiece. We find there a cavity into which we could insert ourselves and fill it with any measure of our excitement.

The family doctor hesitates like one who crosses a river in the winter: respectful as a guest, shimmering like glass in a melting point, simple as uncut wood, as concave as a valley, as formless as the churning water.

Have you not experienced the feeling that in his conversation could only talk about flowers?

# References

http://www.ncbi.nlm.nih.gov/pubmed/26394992.

Okakura K. El libro del té. Barcelona: Editorial Kairós; 1991.

Shin D. Applying the Methodology and Practice of Microhistory: The Diary of a Confucian Doctor, Yi Mun-gŏn (1495-1567). Uisahak. 2015;24(2):389-422.

Turabian JL, Perez Franco B. The wise master or the thirty thousand laws of the four seasons (first part). *Rev Clin Med Fam.* 2013; 6(3). http://www.revclinmedfam.com/articulo.php?pagina=1&art=343.

Turabian JL, Perez Franco B. The wise master or the thirty thousand laws of the four seasons (part 2). *Rev Clin Med Fam.* 2014; 7(1). http://www.revclinmedfam.com/articulo.php?art=350.

Turabian JL, Perez Franco B. The wise master or the thirty thousand laws of the four seasons (last chapter). *Rev Clin Med Fam.* 2014; 7(3). http://www.revclinmedfam.com/articulo.php?art=380.

Turabian JL, Perez Franco B. The wise master, or the thirty thousand laws of the four seasons (part three). *Rev Clin Med Fam.* 2014; 7(2). http://www.revclinmedfam.com/articulo.php?art=367.

Turner-Zwinkels FM, Postmes T, van Zomeren M. Achieving Harmony among Different Social Identities within the Self-Concept: The Consequences of Internalising a Group-Based Philosophy of Life. *PloS One.* 2015; 10(11):e0137879. http://www.ncbi.nlm.nih.gov/pubmed/26618917.

*Chapter 60*

# The Family Doctor as a Tennis Player in a Doubles Match

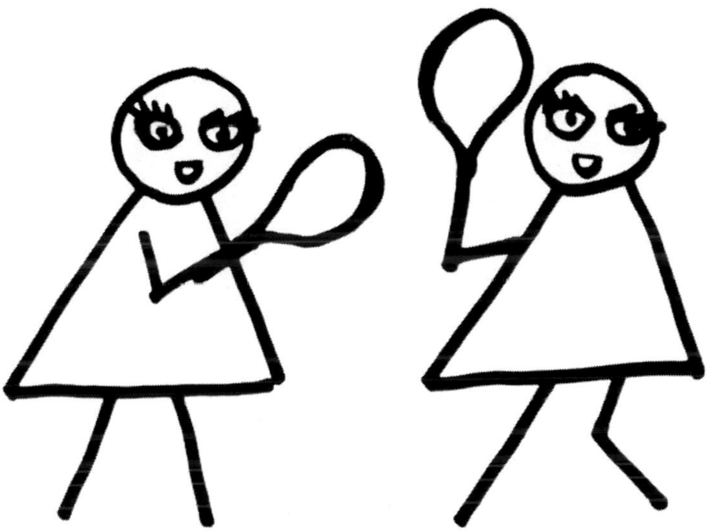

Playing a game of doubles tennis is very different than playing a round of singles tennis. This seems obvious because you is not playing alone, the doubles games requires teamwork and communication, that is, respect, understanding, and constant communication. It is vital to give your partner support and words of encouragement — not individual brilliance but a coordinated collective effort. You must take responsibility to make your partner feel safe, comfortable, and well positioned; moving together. Players feel less pressure because they share the game with their partner and therefore it is often more enjoyable and fun.

If there is a strong player, he must play normally on the side for advantages. If one of the players is very good on the right or the left half of the court he should play in his favored side.

The family doctor usually plays doubles games (or triples, quadruples, etc.!): the patient is also treated by the hospital specialist, the nurse, the social worker, the midwife, the dietician, and so on. The essential rule for the family doctor that is playing a doubles game of tennis is to "respond to the ball player who is best placed in that position" — not the senior one or the one with better qualifications. In many cases, assistance and intervention for the patient can be done for different professionals: it will be done by the person better placed in each particular case.

And always trying to keep positive communication with the other player; keep moving together.

## References

Berman BW. The Generalist–Specialist Interface. Not a Zero-Sum Game. *Clin Pediatr.* 2014; 53(8): 719-20. http://cpj.sagepub.com/content/53/8/719.extract.

Brooks PM. The impact of chronic illness: partnerships with other healthcare professionals. *Med J Aust* 2003; 179 (5): 260-262.

Gallwey WT. The inner game of tennis. New York: Random House; 1974.

http://www.mja.com.au/public/issues/179_05_010903/bro10734_fm.html.

*Chapter 61*

# The Family Doctor as the Painter Giotto

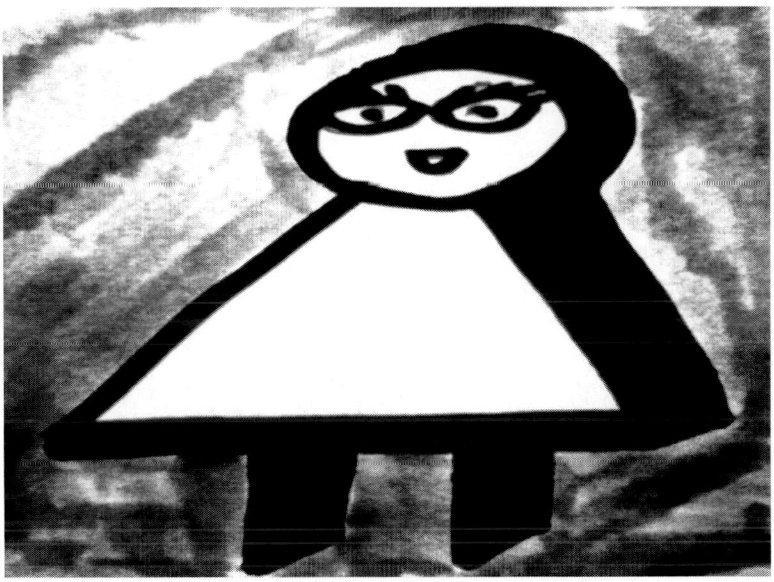

Family doctors are increasingly faced with the presence of multi-morbidity in their patients. Multi-morbidity appears to raise an infinite number of issues and so it is difficult to make useful decisions. How can this multi-morbidity be addressed? What guidelines or protocols are available? Perhaps we could use a qualitative method: the method used by the painter Giotto in his paintings.

Unlike other hospital specialists family doctors use the system that Giotto chose for "highlighting insights" into major problems. These major problems usually remain hidden and can only be unravelled when look at the details.

In his painting Giotto achieved "tactile values," a "third dimension," and a formal approach to visible truths that are configured as material truths about the bi-dimensional plane. He use the contrasts between light and shadow to achieve concave and convex images, and likewise, when the family doctor use this technique, he can see how some problems (health problems) "poke out" in relation to others, giving impression of "strength," making visible the "truth," feeling its "volume," or its "weight," or the family doctor can realizing that he can have a close contact with them, to grasp them, hug them or walking around them.

In his painting, *Polyptych of Badia* (1300), exhibited at the Uffizi, where the Virgin and Child are flanked on the left by St. John the Evangelist and St. Nicholas and on the right by St. Peter and Benedict, which seem"poke out" from surface of painting. In his *Virgin on the throne, Ognissanti Madonna* (circa 1310, also exhibited at the Uffizi, there is a powerful impression of mass relief and solemnity. In his *Funeral of St. Francis* (painted around 1328 and exhibited in Florence in Basilica of Santa Croce, Bardi Chapel), or, for example, in the *Resurrection of the Drusiana believer* (from 1310 to 1320, in the Peruzzi Chapel fresco, of The Santa Croce in Florence), the figures seem to come out of the frame.

Like Giotto, the family doctor uses the qualitative technique of looking holistically at the patient's system and noting that certain problems "poke out" from the rest. These are the problems with "tactile values" or "energy" — all things in the patient's medical history make us look at that particular point, which is highlighted from rest. It is this that gives us a blow to the stomach, which can make heart rate faster, that moves us on many levels, that has a large "density of emotions" — the human elements, the social symbols — and opens up solutions in a patient.

The appearance of solidity, that Giotto had the power to infuse in his works, transforms his two-dimensional configuration of the decorative Gothic tapestries into models with a third dimension. Thus, his figures and architectural elements, which reject any logical perspective, are modelled with such forcefulness that, in the photographic reproduction, with their colors supressed, they appear like sculptural reliefs rather than painting.

The family doctor has to make a workshop in Florence, to learn from Giotto.

## References


Berenson B. The Italian Painters of the Renaissance. Landsmarks in art history. Oxford: Phaidon Press Limited; 1980.

Giotto y la Escuela Florentina. APARENCES. http://www.aparences.net/es/periodos/el-trecento/giotto-y-la-escuela-florentina/.

Los Uffizi. Guía oficial. Florencia: Giunti Editore S.p.A.; 2014.

Sebregondi L. Giotto at Santa Croce. Florencia: Edizioni Polistampa; 2006.

Turabián JL, Pérez Franco B. A way of helping ''Mr. Minotaur'' and ''Ms. Ariadne'' to exit from the multiple morbidity labyrinth: The ''master problems''. Semergen. 2016; 42 (1): 38-48. http://www.elsevier.es/es-revista-semergen-medicina-familia-40-articulo-un-modo-ayudar-al-sr--90447188.

*Chapter 62*

# The Family Doctor as a Sailor

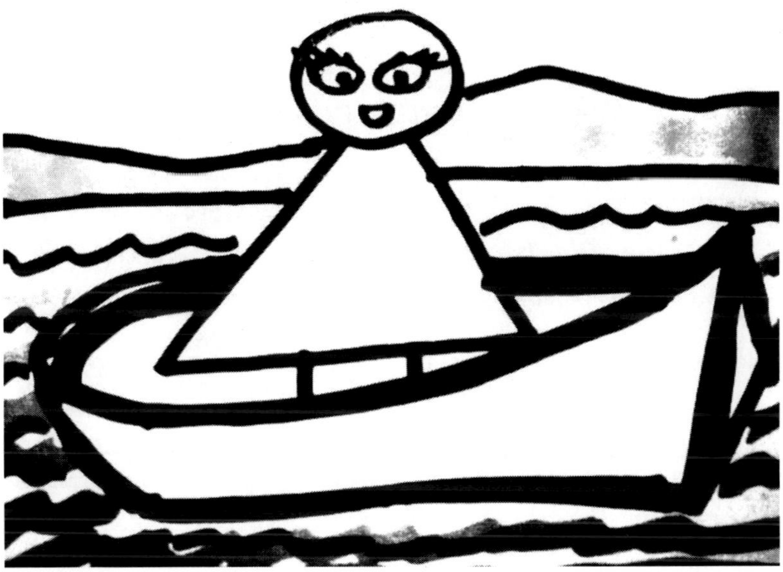

On every trip sailors experience the effect of seeing the earth from sea: at the very moment that man embarks he feels the pleasant sensation of seeing things from a different perspective. From the sea, things on the earth appear to be small and insignificant. The mountains still retain some respectability but the flat areas become a little more or less soft, more or less like thick fog. Villages are surprisingly insignificance once we are half a mile away from them. Houses take assume derisory dimensions and shapes and the roofs and walls soon merge with the earth.

When the family doctor moves away from considering the current query and looks from afar at all the visits of that patient, gets put the current query on your site. Using this technique, like the sailor, the family doctor gets to see key patterns in a nonlinear sequence. Thus, the family doctor can form mental models that utilize the capacity of the entire mind. This facilitates the understanding of the complexity of a problem and allows the connections to become visible, seeing relationships and patterns more clearly. When the family doctor moves "away from the coast and looks from the sea," the situation can be seen in all its dimensions and diagrams can be drawn with a new and clearer view of the situation. “Looking at the coast from the sea allows the doctor to see in the resources and strengths of the family, patterns of events that have been repeated through the generations, family functioning and its relation to events, family structure, coalitions between members, family rules, myths, rituals, and so on.

The family physician seeks to recognize patterns, trends and regularities in a dataset. In these tasks we rely on the ability of physicians, but this is limited by the skills of observation and the analytical tools that are used. In this sense the sea travel is useful, because it helps to put things in its place. “Under insignificant house roofs there are all kinds of minor problems.”

Take the test. Whenever you are in a seaside town try, occasionally, to contemplate the view from a distance of three or four miles. Abandon the narrow streets and porches of the squares. From the sea you will see the amount of nonsense that helps make life unpleasant for men. You will be amazed at the smallness of the things your eyes behold. The view from the sea helps to place the things on land in their proper perspective.

## References

http://www.elsevier.es/es/revistas/atencion-primaria-27/el-concepto-diagnostico-medicina-familia-ver-un-13146911-editorial-2010.

J.L. Turabián, B. Pérez Franco. The diagnostic concept in family medicine: A view of the landscape. The diagnosis in family medicine. *Aten Primaria* 2010;42(2):66-69.

Pla J. Cosas del mar y de la costa brava. Barcelona: Editorial Juventud SA; 1988.

Turabián JL, Pérez Franco B. A way of helping “Mr. Minotaur” and “Ms. Ariadne” to exit from the multiple morbidity labyrinth: The “master problems.” Semergen. 2016; 42(01). http://www.elsevier.es/es-revista-semergen-medicina-familia-40-articulo-un-modo-ayudar-al-sr--90447188.

Turabian JL, Perez Franco B. Family physician’s travel notebook. The sea. *Rev Clin Med Fam.* 2015; 8(1). http://www.revclinmedfam.com/articulo.php?art=404.

*Chapter 63*

# The Family Doctor as a Golfer

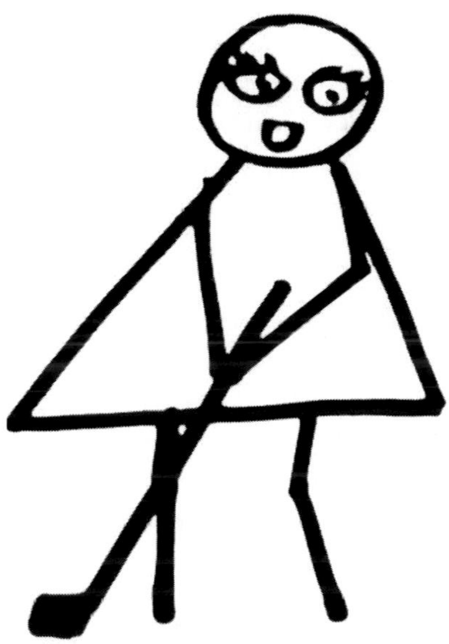

Golf is a sport of precision aimed at using the fewest number of strokes to place a ball into the holes that are distributed in the field. For each type of shot one of a slightly different set of golf clubs is used because the head of the club has different degrees. The golfer is like the family doctor who must resolve the problem — place the ball in the hole — using a limited number of technical skills — the golf clubs.

But there is more, golf entails a lot of mental rather than physical work; analyzing a swing can take about five seconds. A game may last for about four hours although the purely physical part may not be more than five or ten minutes (depending on the number of strokes of each player), which corresponds, more or less, to 5% of the total game time. Indeed, most players spend almost 100% on their physical training part and forget about the mental part.

Family physicians tend to devote 100% of their training time to increasing their knowledge and practical skills, but little or no time in learning how to manage their emotions. Yet, in family medicine, as in golf, improving the latter would not only help us in our game, but also in day-to-day life.

Imagine you are about to play a game of golf — to visit another patient, make a diagnosis, perform a treatment - and you are choosing his favourite brat (choosing between their skills). You feel confident that you will produce a terrific shot, and just then a thought enters your mind: "I mustn't hit the ball into the lake" — "I am unsure about this. What if there is an adverse reaction, kidney failure, that I have overlooked, I do not have enough experience in this." You are suddenly tense, as if frozen. You feel anxiety, stress and fear that the shot might send the ball into the lake. Your mind is interfering ("always shooting into the lake").

Golf is a challenging mental exercise. The thoughts of judgment, over-analysis and self-criticism interfere with your game and enjoyment. You have to empty your mind of these thoughts. Golf is more of a mental exercise than a physical one, but who trains his mind? Currently, the mental control of the game is considered as one of the keys to long-term improvement and to achieving satisfaction from golf. I prefer the term "inner game" involving more than just mental mastery. Sometimes the best thing you can do is to forget the head and trust the body. The mind-body connection has long been investigated and explored in different disciplines, including martial arts, sports, dance, music, art, and medicine, and certainly has a place in golf.

For the golfer and the family doctor discovering and exploring our potential is the key. Once this process begins the true self emerges and the perfect shot is achieved.

The golfer knows the seven principles that will help to increase potential. We apply these principles to family medicine:

1. Be with the feet on the ground, balanced, as if your feet take root in the ground: with calm, relaxed, slow mind; the body in the land, finding your centre.
2. Develop feelings and intuitions; slow down and keep in tune; connect; do what makes you feel good.
3. Be aware of what you want; know what you want; believe in what you want; look to how you can achieve what you want.
4. Create your own ritual for the day or period before an action; find your own space — a place where you feel comfortable; respects your daily ritual.
5. Find your personal natural movement; trust your instincts, listen to your inner voice; find your own way, accept the challenge of making decisions based on your feelings, regardless of others or of negative voices in your head. Focus on what you want. When you trust yourself you can find your way; search your soul.
6. Focus on one thing at a time, even when you have a long list of things to do. Turn off the autopilot. Eliminate distractions and focus on yourself. Clear your mind of other concerns. Each shot is a new beginning. You have to be in that time. Enjoy the moment. Imagine you are in the most beautiful place on earth. Start your ritual, breathe deeply, visualize what you want and just get it; live in the now; surrender to the moment. Do not worry about the past or the future. Focus only on this moment so that you can experience all of your life with awareness. Never miss the moment.
7. Trust the process, take a deep breath and look at the beauty of nature. The great golfers speak of "peace," an experience of peace and serenity. Embrace your journey: when you experience a difficult or inconvenient time look at it as an opportunity to learn and grow. The real beauty is in the moment. That is the most important part of the journey. There is always a calm and peaceful place in a storm. Do not imitate

others; be yourself. Transform your life: change the philosophy of the impossible to the possible. Transform your life by simply putting passion into every aspect of it. Trust the process, take a deep breath and look at the beauty of nature.

## References

Epstein RM. Minful practice. *JAMA*. 1999; 283(9):833–839. http://www.fammed.wisc.edu/files/webfm-uploads/documents/outreach/mindfulness/mindful-practice-epstein.pdf.

Franco C, Justo E. Reducción de los niveles de estrés y ansiedad en médicos de Atención Primaria mediante la aplicación de un programa de entrenamiento en conciencia plena (mindfulness). Aten Primaria. 2010; 42(11):564–570. http://apps.elsevier.es/watermark/ctl_servlet?_f=10&pident_articulo=13184186&pident_usuario=0&pcontactid=&pident_revista=27&ty=86&accion=L&origen=zonadelectura&web=www.elsevier.es&lan=es&fichero=27v42n11a13184186pdf001.pdf.

Gallwey WT. The inner game of golf. London: Pan Books;1979.

Gee D. The seven principles of golf. Mastering the mental game on and off the golf course. New York: Steward, Tabiri & Chang; 2007.

*Chapter 64*

# The Family Doctor as a Filter Coffee

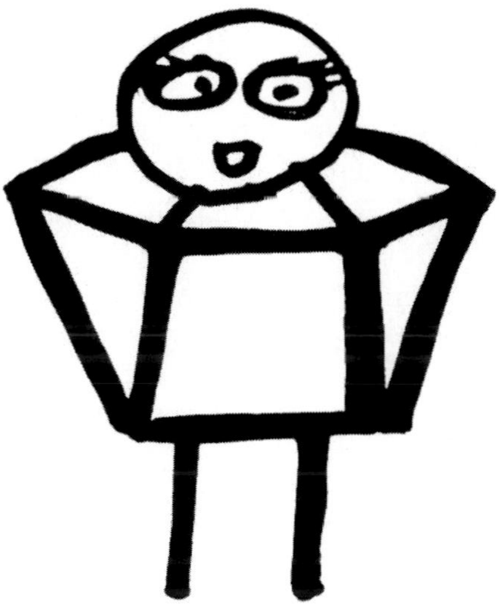

The coffee filter is a kitchen tool that filters the hot water from the coffee grounds. This filter is usually made of paper, which is generally used only once, but there are stainless steel versions. It is the method for making coffee that is most appreciated in the US and northern Europe. It produces an aromatic and flavourful coffee. Coffee percolation was perfected in Germany in the early twentieth century. The grind of the coffee beans is essential: it should be medium. When it is very thick coffee has a weak taste and when it is too fine the taste is bitter. For a good result, the cup coffee should be tasted immediately after preparation.

The utensil that is used to separate the different thickness or screening materials, such as the flour from the bran, is called a sieve. The family doctor has to learn to be like the coffee filter or sieve.

The family doctor has to have the ability to "let go," to forget, or to see the problem as trivial or insignificant and yet, also to keep the recorded medical history in mind — the significant, important, and relevant information. It often happens that what is significant, what makes a diagnosis or prognosis an evolutionary process, is psychological rather than strictly biomedical, and this should encourage the family doctor to pay attention to every part of consultation (which should go through his "coffee filter").

The query by a problem of long date... and precisely today! or a patient with the sad aspect or discouraged... It is not a cold day but the patient is wearing a wool cap covering her hair (scruffy? alopecia?). Her eldest daughter accompanies her and when the doctor asks about the biological symptoms the companion exclaims: "And she will be fired from work!" She says that she plans to retire and want to know where she can ask about her pension. What is significant about this scene? What should the family doctor highlight in the medical record? What elements mark the importance of the diagnosis, the clinical course and prognosis, and treatment? Is this a biomedical diagnosis or an emotional situation entailing work or family?

The filter function of the family doctor saves the patient from the diagnostic and therapeutic excesses of the specialists. Is this smooth coffee? Is this bitter coffee? Would you like a coffee filter?

## References

Gérvas J, Pérez Fernández M. La función de filtro del médico general y el papel de los especialistas en los sistemas de salud. *Rev. Bras. Epidemiol.* 2006; 9 (2). http://www.scielo.br/scielo.php?script=sci_arttext&pid=S1415-790X2006000200012.

Gérvas, J, Pérez Fernández, M. The scientific basis for the gatekeeping role of general practicioners. *Rev Bras Epidemiol.* 2005; 8(2): 205-18. http://equipocesca.org/new/wp-content/uploads/2009/04/filtro-brasil-2005.pdf.

Owens Jaén T. La especialidad de la enfermedad trivial. 2010. http://www.sumaclick.com/owens/la-especialidad/.

Roland M, Coulter A (Editors). Hospital referrals. Oxford: Oxford General Practice Series, 22. Oxford Medical Publications; 1992.

Chapter 65

# The Family Doctor as a Miner

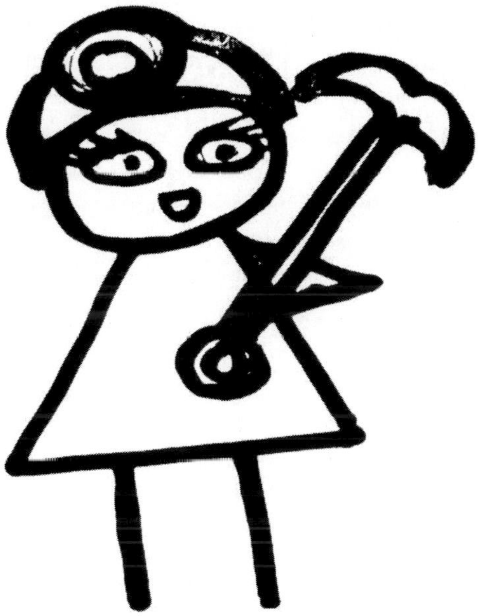

You can dig a mountain to find a vein of precious metals or, more sensibly, you can undertake research to determine exactly where they can be found. Both processes require an immense amount of material.

Over the years, family doctors collect a large amount of bio-psychosocial data on their patients. This results in a database of sufficient size and, if it is of an appropriate quality, the findings are like mining ore in the mine because they provide the doctor with information on patterns and the grouping of concepts that are interesting, potentially useful, and may generate opportunities for research and knowledge.

The family doctor as a miner is faced with great difficulties from the very beginning in that the bottom of the mine is the patient, day after day. To delve into the databases generated by the family doctor we must think with the mind of a miner. The site and all information collected daily is mine is, but it is an unexplored one. To exploit the mine we must find the vein of untapped information.

So, what is the task of mining? Essentially it is to find certain relationships between the objects represented, which would be impossible to find otherwise. What are these relationships? They may be common, yet unexpected features, time sequences, discrepancies or inconsistencies. In addition, new knowledge is the product of the interrelations of all the elements that make up the whole.

The mining a mountain to find a vein of precious metals requires examining a vast amount of material or, more sensibly, investigating more exactly where it might be found.

The most interesting and valuable information relates to the way in which multiple facts interrelate. The work of mining may yield important clues. For the family doctor mining could become a more useful tool for understanding what is happening and trying to visualize the possible paths of a particular sequence of events or to find relationships between seemingly unrelated events. For example, this may entail considering the influences of drug interaction, the characterization and prediction of disease, the likelihood of a satisfactory response to medical treatment, etc.

It is commonly the case that as a result of consultations, diagnosis, complementary tests, interdepartmental referrals and treatments, family physicians generate huge volumes of data but, in the end, produce very little usable and practical information. Similar to a miner who searches tirelessly within a large geological repository of scarce precious metal, the tireless work of the family doctor can produce a tiny nugget of useful information found on a mountain of information slag.

Questions that traditionally required intensive manual analysis can now be answered directly and quickly from the data. Due to time constraints, analysts often have to limit the number of variables they consider when performing manual analysis. However, variables that are discarded because they seem unimportant can provide information about unknown models.

To work as a miner, the family doctor needs to make a "model," i.e., to build a model with features that lead him to a discovery or a hypothesis — a certain definition of variables, but without discarding those that may seem unimportant as they can provide information about strangers. With these models, and with a bit of luck as well, you can find ore.

# References

Bellazzi R, Zupan B.Predictive data mining in clinical medicine: Current issues and guidelines. *International Journal of Medical Informatics.* 2008; 77(2): 81–97. http://core.ac.uk/download/files/382/11678427.pdf.

Qing A, Wei-dong W, Bo-ya Z, Kai-yuan L. Application of data mining based on clinical medicine database. 2010 2nd International Conference on Signal Processing Systems (ICSPS); Volume:3: V3-719 - V3-723. http://ieeexplore.ieee.org/xpl/login.jsp?tp=&arnumber=5555754&url=http%3A%2F%2Fieeexplore.ieee.org%2Fxpls%2Fabs_all.jsp%3Farnumber%3D5555754.

Amarasingham R, Moore BJ, Tabak YP, Drazner MH, Clark CA, Zhang S, et al. An automated model to identify heart failure patients at risk for 30-day readmission or death using electronic medical record data. *Medical Care.* 2010 48: 981- 988. http://www.ncbi.nlm.nih.gov/pubmed/20940649.

Soler JK, Corrigan D, Kazienko P, Kajdanowicz T, Danger R, Kulisiewicz M, et al. Evidence-based rules from family practice to inform family practice; the learning healthcare system case study on urinary tract infections. BMC Family Practice. 201516:63. http://bmcfampract.biomedcentral.com/articles/10.1186/s12875-015-0271-4.

Dávila Hernández F, Sánchez Corales IY. Data mining techniques aplied to diagnosys of clinical entities. *Revista Cubana de Informática Médica.* 2012; 4(2). http://scielo.sld.cu/scielo.php?script=sci_arttext&pid=S1684-18592012000200007.

*Chapter 66*

# The Family Doctor as a Tailor

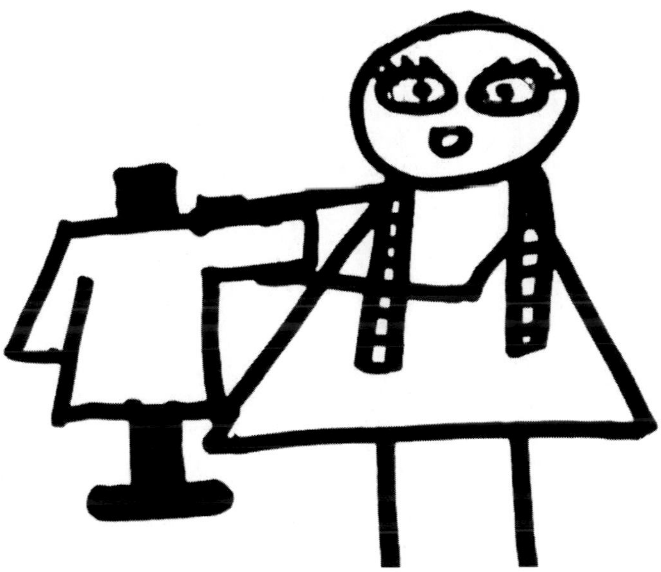

If I wanted a suit that would fit like a glove, what would I do? I would go to a tailor to take my measurement. A tailor makes a suit to fit a person and he uses the available fabrics. So, the family doctor has to varying his treatments for "fit" with the specific resources of the person. The experience of having a tailored suit is very special, it makes us feel safe, powerful, and elegant, but it is particularly special because it is something that was chosen for us and made for our body, the use of which results in great comfort.

The family doctor has a lot to learn from the tailor: tailored suits for his patients by "taking the measurements" of each particular patient, and knowing his particular needs and perspectives. One of the most common errors committed in family medicine is to provide "the same operation or the same advice to everyone." But, it is quite obvious that it is not possible to individualize all interventions. Yet, it is done. So it is that the family doctor, believing that some intervention or advice was appropriate for a particular patient, extrapolates this to other patients. If we also add that it is always easier to use a single technique than to use many, we have a set routine.

That is one reason why the family doctor as a therapist has to make "suits." In general, several or many consultations are needed with the patient to discover their needs, personality, and all those characteristics that define us in terms of how we think and act most of the time. The family doctor should discover the characteristics of the real self of the patient in order to "take measurements."

Most people are unaware that there are so many things that can be measured in our bodies. A woman's shirt requires some seventeen different measurements. The tailor accurately takes these measurements. Just the act being measured is something that everyone should experience: it is something gratifying and rewarding; and it takes time.

The best thing about the tailor's method of work is to realize that what lead to neurosis for one person is healing for another. To take an example, there are some very hard-working and demanding people that need relax, be less exigent to themselves and do less. Instead, there are very self-indulgent people who need to be activated and be a little more exigent to themselves. So there are no useful standards that fit everyone, each approach depends on the nature of the patient.

If family physicians want to find interventions that make the patient feel good, the first thing they have to do is to "take her measurements" or, in other words, to know the particular patient well. Only when the family doctor has that information can the pattern be properly designed: the health plan to help the particular patient; a tailored suit produced for each patient.

# References

Chen J, Mullins CD, Novak P, Thomas SB.Personalized Strategies to Activate and Empower Patients in Health Care and Reduce Health Disparities. *Health Educ Behav.* 2016; 43(1): 25-34. http://heb.sagepub.com/content/43/1/25?etoc.

Jakovljević M, Ostojić L. Person-centered medicine and good clinical practice: disease has to be cured, but the patient has to be healed. *Psychiatr Danub.* 2015;27 Suppl 2:546-9. http://www.ncbi.nlm.nih.gov/pubmed/26657982.

Krahn M. 'New' Evidence for Clinical Practice Guidelines: Should We Search for 'Preference Evidence'? *The Patient - Patient-Centered Outcomes Research.* 2010; 3(2):71-77. http://rd.springer.com/journal/40271.

Métter I. La quinta esquina. Barcelona: Libros del asteroide; 2014.

Neighbourg R. The inner consultation. Lancaster: *MTP press*, 1991.

No place for "one size fits all" in Scots schools. *Scottish Government.* 23/05/2002. http://www.scotland.gov.uk/pages/news/2002/05/SEED024.aspx.

Chapter 67

# The Family Doctor as a Diver

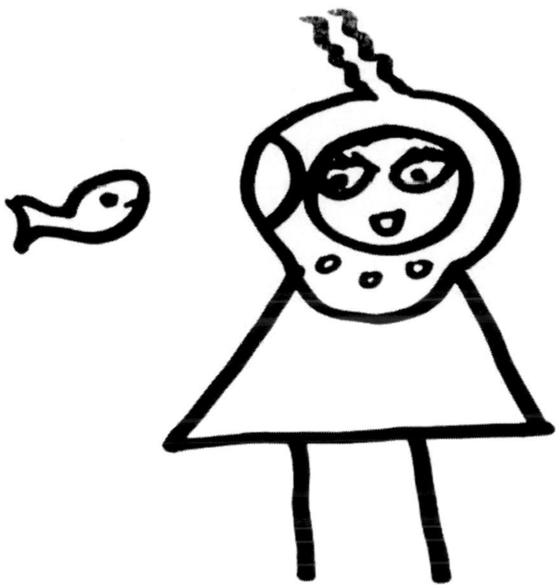

The family doctor sees only a portion of the patient's health problems: the ones that he talks about so that the doctor can define or diagnose. But all family physician know that most of the problems remain hidden. These are like an iceberg, a large mass of floating ice whose top protrudes from the surface of the sea, which is all we see. Of course, the emotional and psychosocial dimensions of biological diseases are the aspects that are often in the hidden part of the iceberg and, therefore, are frequently overlooked when considering medical intervention.

So, the family doctor needs to be like a diver, a person who performs tasks when submerged in water. Using special equipment the diver descend underwater and explores the great hidden base of the iceberg. In addition, according to the family doctor/diver the more you descend below the surface of the water, the more complex are the problems encountered!

For example, the tip of the iceberg may be a patient with uncomplicated angina pectoris or cluster headache. When we descend to the unseen area, we can note that the same patient is of a low social class with angina, cluster headache, depression and alcohol abuse, which also presents legal, economic, and family problems. If we continue the descent, we can see the same patient with acute intoxication as a result of excessive consumption of alcohol, with angina, depression, and cluster headache. This patient is a smoker who lives in an isolated rural area and has legal, economic, family, and religious problems, which, by default, lead to frequent consultations with occasionally hostile behavior. At the tip of the iceberg the patient could have been considered an "easy case" but examining the base reveals that it to be "a very difficult case"!

Of course, it is a mistake to rank thus the clinical cases because this classification is conventional and useful only for educational purposes: all problems are always complex but are qualified as such depending on where our inquiry arbitrarily stops. It depends on how far down we dive!

## References

http://www.elsevier.es/es/revistas/semergen-medicina-general--familia-40/un-caso-facil-o-dificil-las-formas-13184353-editorial-2010.

Last JM. The iceberg: "completing the clinical picture" in general practice. *The Lancet* 1963; 282 (7297): 28 - 31. http://www.lancet.com/journals/lancet/article/PIIS0140-6736(63)92546-7/fulltext.

Smith GD- Are there 'social causes' of mortality? *Int. J. Epidemiol.* 2015; 44 (5):1493-1495. http://ije.oxfordjournals.org/content/44/5/1493.extract?etoc.

Turabian JL, Perez Franco B. An easy or difficult case? Shapes drawn from life. Uncertainty based family medicine. Medicina de familia basada en la incertidumbre. *Semergen* 2010;36(9):485-490.

*Chapter 68*

# The Family Doctor as a Poet

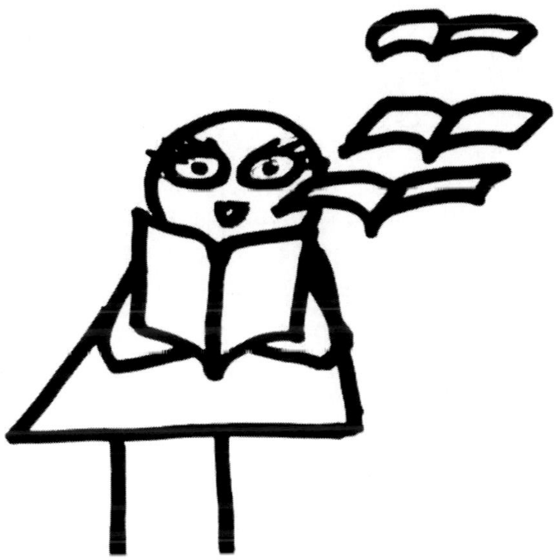

There are many paths to climb in the attainment of knowledge. It seems, however, that over the last century the dominant approach in Western thought has only recognized the Cartesian positivist paradigm as a valid the process for gaining knowledge.

Poetry is a form of knowledge. Different types of problems require different types of knowledge. Poetry can be a source of knowledge by providing us with perspectives of reality, and in this sense it can also have a cognitive impact on us and on our understanding of the world.

The prevailing belief in a measurable and deterministic truth has begun to disappear. We now accept that there are many forms of knowledge. Life, in its constant expansion and creativity, including uncertainty, provides us with open-ended, unwritten experiences, with changes and surprises. Thus, uncertainty is an essential element in human existence.

The family doctor, in contrast to the hospital doctor, is most often occupied in taking decisions in an environment of complex and chaotic systems where quantitative, evidence-based medicine and evidence-based guidelines — protocols, guides, clinical knowledge —

are not enough. Thus, the family doctor should use other scientific paradigms and other vague rules to address problems where traditional methods are of little use.

Family medicine is the art of working with uncertainty and creativity. The family doctor has to learn to live with uncertainty, which is the question that professionals have to consider in terms of the correctness of their clinical decisions or the results that are obtained from them. The tolerance for uncertainty requires the ability to receive a great deal of conflicting information without forcing the situation, and to maintain an internal locus of evaluation.

Doubts can become a good quality if you can use them carefully. Doubt has to become wisdom; it has become critical. The family doctor has to ask the question, ask for tests, and submit to examination. The doubt may be perplexing and bewildering, perhaps even irritating. But the family doctor should not give in. Ask for reasons to doubt!

The family doctor must have patience with what is still not resolved and must try to love the questions themselves, like locked rooms or books written in a strange language. "Do not look now for the answers: they cannot be given, because you could not live with them."

To act with confidence you should be able to look ahead and consider uncertainties. You should not devote too much time to considering distant possibilities; the key is to find the significant one. But important questions about the future are generally too complex or imprecise for the conventional language of science. Rather than using this language we should used poetic language, which has a psychological impact that the equations and graphs lack.

Obtaining knowledge is not a simple phenomenon. It occurs in a somewhat labyrinthine manner amid countless secondary phenomena of acceleration, condensation, regression or survival; and is a discontinuous phenomenon whose successive moments may be separated by long periods.

Therefore, family physicians have to use the methods of obtaining knowledge and to face the uncertainty of consultation that is used by poets.

## References

Campo R. The poetry of healing. New York: W. W. Norton & Company; 1997.

Camus A. El mito de Sísifo. Madrid: Alianza Editorial S.A.; 1995.

http://journals.lww.com/academicmedicine/Fulltext/2011/07000/Commentary__Ambiguity_and_Uncertainty__Neglected.7.aspx.

http://www.amazon.co.uk/Cuadernos-medicina-familia-y-comunitaria/dp/8479781920.

Luther VP, Crandall SJ. Commentary: Ambiguity and Uncertainty: Neglected Elements of Medical Education Curricula? Academic Medicine. 2011; 86 (7):799-800.

Rilke RM. Cartas a un joven poeta. Barcelona: ediciones obelisco, S.L.; 1986.

Rof Carballo J. Entre el silencio y la palabra. Madrid: Colección Austral. Espasa Calpe; 1990.

Turabian JL. Cuadernos de Medicina de Familia y Comunitaria. Una introducción a los principios de Medicina de Familia. Madrid: Díaz de Santos. 1995.

Chapter 69

# The Family Doctor as a Philosopher

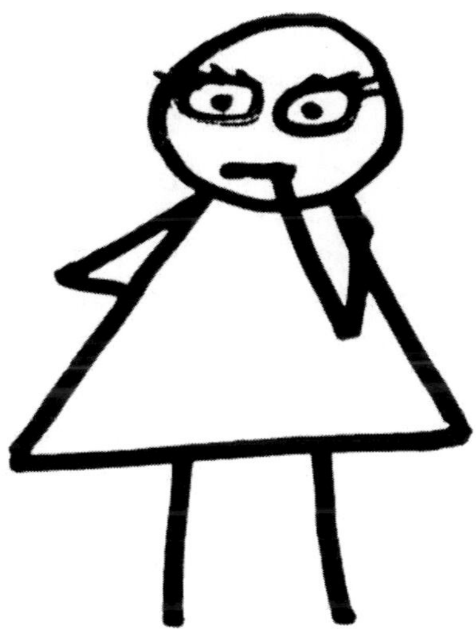

Philosophers can present us with new ideas that are grounded in the great traditions of human thought. Philosophical expertise encompasses logic, ethics, values, meanings, rationality, and decision-making in conflicting or risky situations, in short, all the immense complexity that characterizes human life. Epicurus said that, "against the diseases of the mind, philosophy has remedies."

In all fairness, philosophy can be seen as the medicine of the mind. Philosophy can be useful in providing sets of knowledge for healing individual and social pathologies in the post-industrial world that besets mankind. There is an increasing number of people who live in rich countries with seemingly settled lives and yet they experience endless problems in their personal and professional lives that constantly embitter them. What many people need is dialogue, not a diagnosis.

Family physicians need to help patients to think critically, seeking patterns of behavior and then placing them in the broader context of their way in life. Understanding the patient's own philosophy can help you to avoid many of the problems that need to be addressed or resolved. The philosophy of the patient may also be the source of the problems he has, thus the physician and the family must evaluate the ideas that sustain patients to model a point of view that to be in our favour, not against. With the help of the "philosopher" patients may be able to change the patients to model a point of view that to be in our favour, not against. their beliefs in order to solve the problem.

With the patient, the philosopher can discuss Kierkegaard's approach to facing death, Ayn Rand's ideas about the virtues of selfishness, or Aristotle's advice to pursue reason and moderation in all things, the theory of taking decisions of the I Ching (Book of Changes), or Kant's theory of needs. Depending on the patient's problem, the "philosopher" examines the ideas that best apply to the case, those with which the patient can feel more comfortable. Patients may prefer the authoritarian approach of Hobbes, for example, whereas others may respond to more intuitive approaches, such as those of Lao Tse. The "philosopher" will explore these philosophies in depth, but most likely it will be that the patient with his own philosophical scheme who wants to express it more clearly. Here the "philosopher" act as a guide to uncover and illuminate their own ideas and, possibly, to suggest new ones.

The work of the family doctor as a philosopher is to help people understand what kind of problems they face and, through dialogue, to disentangle and classify the components and implications, thus assisting them to find the best solutions. A philosophical approach that is compatible with his own belief system and at the same time, in line with principles enshrined of wisdom, that contributes to lead a virtuous life and effective.

One moment where it can be especially helpful for the family doctor to act as a philosopher is during the clinical interview. The first requirement is to identify the problem. We usually know when we have a problem as most of us have an internal alarm mechanism that goes off when we need help or additional resources. There are times when we realize that the problem is more complicated, so this stage can take some effort. Each of us is cantered in our own being and sees the world from a strategic position. We can perceive of existence as a mere series of events that happen to us and around us, or we can assume some responsibility for many of the things that happen. Usually we accept responsibility for the positive developments and we remain aloof from the negative ones.

When patients are ready to define the problems they face, family doctor should seek to find out what happens without judgment. It is to see what philosophers call "phenomena," i.e., events that are external to oneself, facts that exist independently of beliefs, feelings or desires. Usually people handle the most routine situations and we have to examine every new state of things because we have social conventions and personal habits to guide us. Thus, when analyzing the situation the patient has to determine what a new phenomenon is and what the real problem is for him.

Subsequently, an internal and external accounting process needs to be undertaken. Here, an important aspect is that the customer must gather the emotions that cause the problem. You should experience genuine emotions and channel them constructively. The patient's emotions can be a combination of grief, anger and sadness, but perhaps it will require some effort for the patient to reach this conclusion.

These first two stages frame the issue and most people go through them naturally and may not need anyone to help them identify the problem, but this is not always the case. In analyzing the patient the process of solving the problem begin by carrying out an inventory of the options and available resources.

Finally, after stating the problem and expressing their emotions, the options have to be weighed and the situation viewed from a holistic approach, one that will reach equilibrium.

The patient understands the essence of the problem and is ready to take appropriate and justifiable acts. He will feel balanced and ready to face the inevitable changes ahead.

Some people are able to cover the four stages in a single consultation or counselling session; for others the process may weeks, months or years. The amount of time necessary for consultations will vary depending on the patient and the situation. Some patients have already gone through the first three stages (identifying the problem, analyzing the emotions and examining the options) prior to consulting the doctor. Where this is the case, the process continues from where the patient is at and must proceed at their pace.

## References


Lou Marinoff. Más Platón y menos Prozac. Ediciones B; 2000.

Rogers CR. On becoming a person. Boston: Houghton Mifflin Company; 1961.

Turabian JL, Perez Franco B. Entrevista clínica participativa-capacitadora: otra alternativa para las consultas de la Sra. Pesáez. FMC 2000;7(7):491-492.

Turabián JL. Innovaciones en metodología docente. El aprendizaje capacitador. JANO, Medicina y Humanidades. 2000;1328 (58): 11.

Wompner F, Fernández Montt R. Aprender a aprender. Un método valioso para la educación superior. Observatorio de la Economía Latinoamericana. Revista académica de economía. 2007. http://www.eumed.net/cursecon/ecolat/cl/2007/fwrf-aprender.htm.

Yalom ID. Un año con Schpenhauer. Buenos Aires: Emecé Editores S.A.; 2006.

*Chapter 70*

# The Family Doctor as a Billiards Player

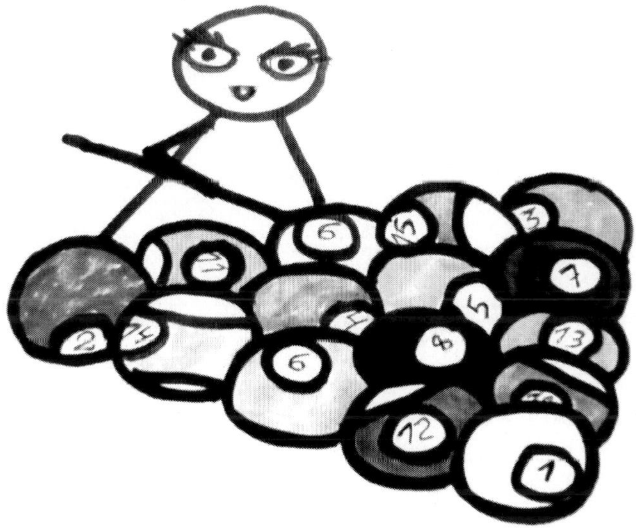

Pool is a popular form of billiards. In this game there are typically 15 balls and the table has 6 holes, four in the corners and two more in the centre of each long side of the table. The balls must be potted into these holes following the specific rules of the game. The balls hit each other and in turn push others. The way in which a ball is struck by another ball will determine the direction of travel. Multiple blows between the balls and their different direction of travel means that other ball may be hit.

Similarly, human behavior cannot be explained solely in linear and individual terms. The family environment or context is relevant to understanding the behavior of its members in the same way that the balls on a pool table are affecting through their contact with each other. Disease cannot be seen as a property of the individual but as a product of the interaction of individuals with their context.

The theory learned by the family doctor is systemically applied to the family in a similar way to watching the game of billiards. What are traditionally called individual, family and community cares are elements of the same reality and cannot be separated: that is, there is no individual attention; rather, it is always attention to the family and the community over time.

When properly attending to a person, we are undertaking individual, family and community care at the same time. All health problems are simultaneously bio-psychosocial, individual, group and community issues.

The context includes the pathology, the illness, the person and the environment. Each person is part of multiple, interconnected systems that include the family, the ethnic group, colleagues, social contacts, work and school environments, and religion. Clinical care, health promotion, disease prevention, and health education need to take account of the context.

The doctor-patient relationship is actually triangular: doctor-patient-family. The family doctor has to be aware that some actors impact on the positions of others. We have to take the family as the primary point for directing our treatment (hygienic measures, diet, taking medication, exercise, rest, and so on). We also have to take into account the "impact" that occurs between family members and how others are "moved" by it. When a subsystem (which can be biological, individual, family, community, etc.) is hit, this affects the others, both in terms of health and disease. The family has an important influence on health: asthma, cardiovascular disease, hypertension, obesity, mental health, infections, physician visits, and hospital admissions.

The more complex the problem to be addressed, the more work we need to do with the family. To conceive of the family as a system helps us to understand the individual symptoms that may have a role in family dynamics. The persistence of symptoms may indicate a difficulty in a particular family situation that needs to be changed or that needs to address a particular conflict.

## References

Camus A. La peste. Barcelona: Pocket Edasa; 1998.

Cogswell BE, Sussman MB (Editors). Family Medicine: A new approach to health care. New York: The Haworth Press; 1982.

Rolland JS. Families, illness, and disability. An integrative treatment model. New York: Bassic Books; 1994.

Srivastava R. Complicated Lives — taking the social history. *N Engl J Med* 2011; 365:587-589. http://www.nejm.org/doi/pdf/10.1056/NEJMp1106985.

Turabian JL, Pérez Franco B. Actividades comunitarias en medicina de familia y atención primaria. Madrid: Díaz de Santos; 2001.

Turabián JL, Pérez Franco B. modelos de atención centrada en el "acompañante" del paciente. La familia y el contexto: en el borde de la relación médico-paciente en medicina de familia. Berlin: Editorial Académica Española. Schaltungsdienst Lange o.H. G.; 2015. https://www.morebooks.de/store/es/book/modelos-de-atenci%C3%B3n-centrada-en-el-acompa%C3%B1ante-del-paciente/isbn/978-3-659-09775-1.

Turabián JLl, Pérez franco B. The Doctor With Three Heads. Aten Primaria. 2006;38(10):570-3. http://www.elsevier.es/es-revista-atencion-primaria-27-articulo-el-medico-tres-cabezas-13095929.

*Chapter 71*

# The Family Doctor as Sancho Panza

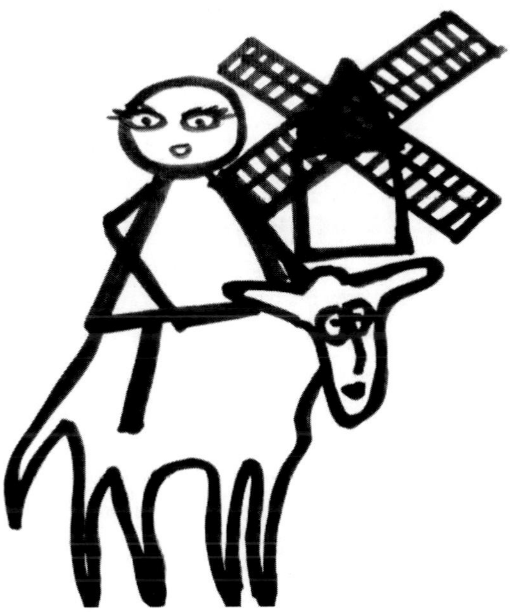

Sancho Panza is one of the fictional characters in the novel *The Ingenious Hidalgo Don Quixote* written by Miguel de Cervantes. Don Quixote, the main character is a knight who decides to go off in search of adventure. Tradition dictates that every knight has a squire. Thus, Don Quixote convinces Sancho Panza, a farmer who was his neighbor, to be his squire. If the real protagonist is Don Quixote, standing beside him is the beloved figure his squire Sancho Panza.

Unlike Don Quixote Sancho Panza is a realistic and practical man who faithfully follows his knight even though he does not understand his idealism. While Don Quixote is dedicated to undoing imaginary wrongs, for his part, Sancho is a simple and good-natured man who tries to prevent Don Quixote from getting into difficult situations. Don Quixote looks like a madman who distorts reality and whose behavior places him in danger. Sancho Panza is a mixture of ingenuity and wit, which gives him credibility and originality. Throughout the novel Sancho demonstrates his sanity and his enriched humanity.

In the adventure with the windmills, Don Quixote imagines that these windmills are giants and he is determined to fight them. This applies to situations where the person fights for a goal or an ideal, often taking on an indefinite and inaccessible "enemy" with little chance of success. Sancho immediately warned him that these were not giants but windmills. Don Quixote is thrown by the blades of the windmill and he falls to the ground with his broken spear. Sancho Panza helps him up and leads him through the path avoiding further blows from the blades of the windmills. Later in the novel, two friars appear on their mules and Don Quixote immediately mistakes them for witches. He was ready to attack. Sancho advised him to avoid greater evils, just as he did with the windmills.

The family doctor is like Sancho Panza. Patients engage in risky behaviors and have physical and mental health problems. Often the doctor cannot solve or change those circumstances. If the family doctor cannot cure the patient, the doctor should at least do no harm and should avoid creating more suffering for the patient. Curing may entail doing nothing. When the patient is terminally ill, there are times when it is better to do nothing, just be there. The necessary skills required here are medical intuition, compassion, knowing our limits, and using courage and integrity.

A treatment may "accompany" the patient to avoid more risks and traumas, as Sancho Panza did for Don Quixote.

# References

Cassell EJ. *The Nature of Suffering and the Goals of Medicine*. Oxford: Oxford University Press; 1991.

Com acompanyar fins a la mort. Document del grup d´ètica de la CAMFIC. 2 de març de 2012. http://metgedefamilia.blogspot.com/2012/03/com-acompanyar-fins-la-mort.html.

de Cervantes Saavedra M. El ingenioso hidalgo Don Quijote de la Mancha. Ciudad de la Habana. Editorial Arte y Literatura. Biblioteca de Literatura Universal; 1989.

M. Ayarra, S. Lizarraga. Bad news and emotional support. ANALES Sis San Navarra 2001; 24 (Supl. 2): 55-63. http://docplayer.es/13803280-Malas-noticias-y-apoyo-emocional-bad-news-and-emotional-support.html.

Ortiz A, Beca JP, Salas SF, Browne F, Salas C. Accompanying a patient as an experience to learn the meaning of disease. Rev Méd Chile 2008; 136: 304-309. http://www.scielo.cl/scielo.php?script=sci_arttext&pid=S0034-98872008000300004&lng=en&nrm=iso&ignore=.html.

Turabian fernandez JL. Una medicina a escala humana. JANO 2003; LXV(1489):10. http://www.jano.es/ficheros/sumarios/1/65/1489/10/1v65n1489a13052086pdf001.pdf.

*Chapter 72*

# The Family Doctor as a Candle Light

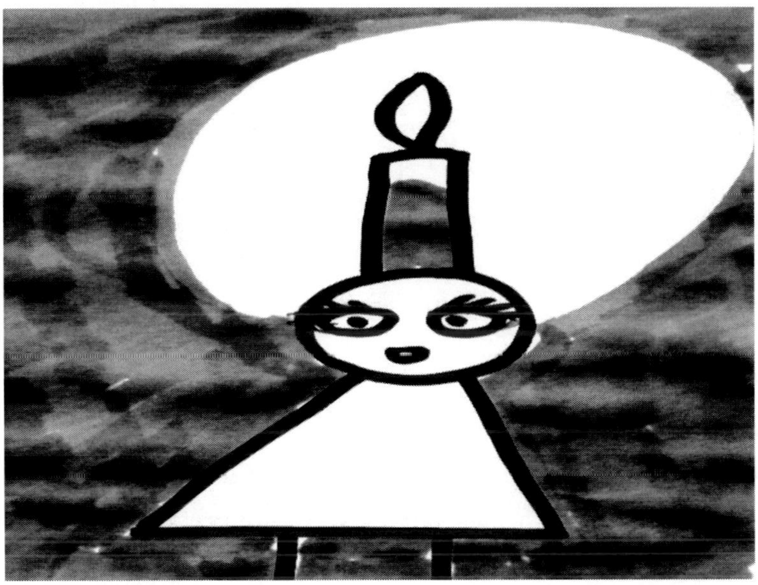

Initiating a medical treatment is like providing the patient with a therapeutic "light." But to avoid dazzling the patient with techniques or interventions the light must not be too bright. The role of the family doctor is to illuminate because there are differences between "light" and "dazzling light"; light is to deepen oneself; dazzle is to do hasty and thunderous gestures. A candle or a lamp gives light that allows you to see better whereas dazzling lights blind and impede vision. Very new products run the risk of producing glare, the glare that might result, for example, in adverse reactions to new drugs.

Family physicians can have therapeutic inertia that produces highly inappropriate, dangerous, and expensive polypharmacy, partly because of the requirements coming from the hospital level, but also the result of the glare of family doctors themselves, doctors who are responsible for a substantial amount of all initial prescriptions for new medicines. In this way doctors are forgetting the therapeutic role of shedding "light" rather than "dazzling" their patients.

Judicious, cautious and conservative prescription, illuminating but not dazzling, is a prerequisite for the safe and proper use of medications, and this includes scepticism about new drugs, and the maintenance of surveillance for adverse reactions.

## References

Báez-Montiel BB, Gutiérrez-Islas E, Herrera-Ontañón JR, Turabián JL. Iluminar y deslumbrar. Un caso de prescripción inadecuada de prasugrel con reacción adversa urticante. *Aten Primaria.* 2013;45:64-5.

http://zl.elsevier.es/es/revista/atencin-primaria-27/articulo/iluminar-deslumbrar-un-caso-prescripcion-90185340?referer=buscador.

Ruiz-Moral R, Parras-Rejano JM, Alcalá-Partera JA, Castro-Martín E, Pérula de Torres LA. Wellcome and i´ll see you again or hello and goodbye?: communicative behaviour of medical residents in the first and last moments of consultations. *Aten Primaria* 2005; 36: 537 – 541. http://apps.elsevier.es/watermark/ctl_servlet?_f=10&pident_articulo=13082486&pident_usuario=0&pcontactid=&pident_revista=27&ty=131&accion=L&origen=zonadelectura&web=www.elsevier.es&lan=es&fichero=27v36n10a13082486pdf001.pdf.

Sampedro JL. Escribir es vivir. Barcelona: Debolsillo; 2007.

*Chapter 73*

# The Family Doctor as a Mother Who Picks Up Her Baby

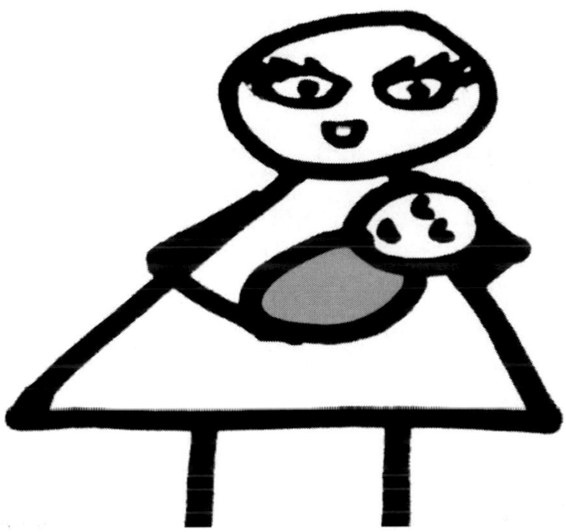

The instruments used by the family doctor — the stethoscope, otoscope, reflex hammer, sphygmomanometer — are not so much a set of instruments to examine the body as a tool to make contact. This human contact may occur in a moment or may never be instituted at all.

The family doctor should maintain a type of connection with the patient that is "here, right now, at this specific moment." This is similar to a mother who learns not to take her baby into her arms when it cries but, rather, to maintain a connection with the crying baby. A baby can discern whether the arms that hold it are clenched in anger or just trying to control it, or are simply open and willing to be with the baby. If the arms are angry and trying to control, the baby will fight sleep. When the mother's arms are relaxed and open, the baby will sleep.

Thus, the family doctor sees patients in new ways. It is not only his words but also something else, everything around him and everything in the space that develops between the patient and the physician, just as in the field in the summer where you can almost see the breeze ruffling the wheat. So it can happen that a patient suffering, although at that time was talking cheerfully, we may feel his pain so intensely that we begin to have tears in our eyes.

The question that the family doctor needs to ask to achieve that connection is, "Can we try to understand, you and me together?" This gives rise to the "click" or "flash" that creates the environment for advancing the diagnosis and treatment.

# References

Balint E, Norell JS (Ed). Six minutes for the patient: interactions in general practice consultations. London: Tavistock publications; 1973.

Buckman R. Communications and emotions. *BMJ* 2002;325:672. http://www.bmj.com/content/325/7366/672.full.

Hesse H. En el balneario. Barcelona. Primera Plana S.A.; 1993.

Shem S. Monte Miseria. Barcelona: Editorial Anagrama; 2000.

Turabian JL, Perez Franco B. The Effect of Seeing the Sea for the First Time. An Attempt at Defining the Family Medicine Law: The Interview is Clinical Medicine. Aten Primaria 2008; 40(11):565-566. http://www.elsevier.es/es/revistas/atencion-primaria-27/el-efecto-ver-primera-vez-mar-un-13128570-reflexiones-medicina-familia-2008.

*Chapter 74*

# The Family Doctor as a Nuts and Bolts Mechanism

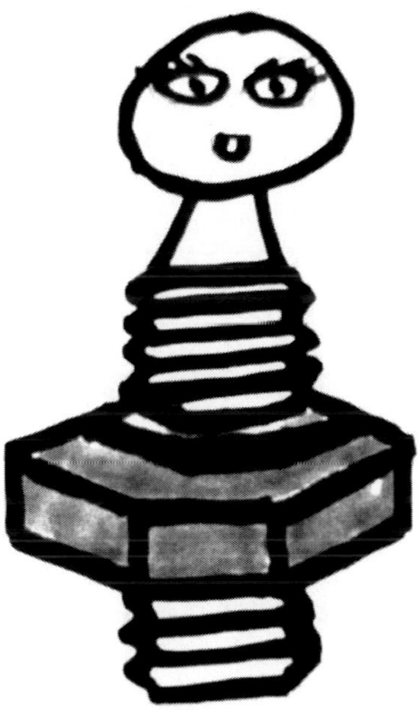

In the nut and bolt mechanism, the nut moves with a rectilinear movement outside the screw. The circular nut movement becomes a linear movement that imprisons the object between the screw and the nut. It is a cycle that moves the nut. The family doctor uses a similar learning mechanism in family medicine: the reflection-action cycle.

The formative period of the family doctor is a critical step in the development of professional identity because learned habits extend beyond those formative years. Patterns are forged in response to stress and work intensity. Unfortunately, on many occasions there is a mismatch between personal and professional development habits. These problems are common during this period of training: stress, information overload, time of work, responsibility and autonomy, as well as new working relationships with patients, nurses, administrative personnel, doctors, other residents and family life.

Furthermore, doctors have to recognize their lack of experience and the mistakes that they may make. During these early days of training it may be the case that there is no substantial learning of the bio-psychosocial model, and doctors in training have little time or incentive to care about the doctor-patient-family relationship. A simple alternative to prevent the development of maladaptive behavior modes is to facilitate a process of reflection and action. This cycle is like the nut that screws onto the screw. The family physician training begins, individually or in groups, and this leads him to a gradual process of personal and professional reflection. Moving within this cycle or nut-screw mechanism, as the nut turns on the bolt, increasingly tightens the object and each time knowledge and skills are improved.

From the concrete experience, to the reflection and analysis of the experience, the identification of theoretical frameworks to explain the experience and, finally, its implementation through active experimentation, effectively integrate new learning and consequently, over time, they consolidate, develop, and refine knowledge, skills and attitudes.

## References

De Bono E. *Practical thinking*. London: Penguin Books; 1976.

Flew A. Thinking about Thinking. Glasgow: William Collins Sons & Co.; 1985.

García Huete E. Aprender a pensar bien. Madrid: Santillana SA; 1998.

http://www.elsevier.es/es/revistas/atencion-primaria-27/mapas-aventura-13118069-cartas-al-director-2008.

Mamede, S. and Schmidt, H. G. (2004), The structure of reflective practice in medicine. *Medical Education,* 38: 1302–1308. http://onlinelibrary.wiley.com/doi/10.1111/j.1365-2929.2004.01917.x/abstract.

Marañón G. El dogmatismo médico y la Medicina antidogmática.En: La Medicina de nuestro tiempo. Madrid: Espasa Calpe, SA; 1980.

Shah I. Learning how to learn. New York; Penguin Books Inc; 1983.

Shah T. El aprendiz de brujo. Madrid: Alba Editorial; 2000.

Turabian Fernandez JL, Perez Franco B. *Map Towards Adventure.* Aten Primaria 2008;40(4):209-216.

# Authors' Contact Information


***Dr. José Luis Turabian***
Medico de Familia
Tutor de Residentes
Centro de Salud Poligono Industrial
SESCAM
Toledo. España.
Calderon de la Barca, 24, Yepes, Toledo, Spain
jturabianf@hotmail.com

***Dr. Benjamin Perez-Franco***
Specialist in Family and Community Medicine
Health Center "The Station"
Talavera de la Reina. SESCAM
Toledo,Spain.

# Index

## D

## E



## F

## G



## H



## I

## N



## O



## P

## T



## U

## V



## W



## Y